HEALTH

Decluttering The Natural Health Industry & Rethinking Chronic Disease

Dr. Robert W. Horovitz, B.Sc., ND

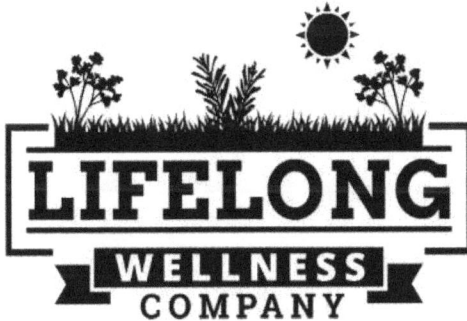

LIFELONG
WELLNESS
COMPANY

Robert W. Horovitz
647-268-4869
robert@lifelongwell.ca
www.lifelongwell.ca
Instagram @roberthorovitz

Publisher: The Lifelong Wellness Company

Disclaimer

This book contains information that is intended to help the readers be better informed consumers of health care. It is presented as general advice on health care. Always consult your doctor for your individual needs. Before beginning any new exercise, nutritional (including herbs and supplements) intervention, or wellness program it is recommended that you seek medical advice from your personal physician. This book is not intended to be a substitute for the medical advice of a licensed physician. The reader should consult with their doctor in any matters relating to his/her health.

Dedication

This book along with my life's work in helping people is dedicated to my parents Evelin and Eitan Horovitz who taught me the meaning of true, unconditional love and life, and who always have and continue to inspire me every day for the rest of the days of my life. You have given me the gift of gab, a noble sense of trying to do the right thing, and a sense of how awesome life truly is. You are the absolute reason why I thirst úor lifelong wellness. As well, to my grandparents Rebecca Horovitz, Abraham Horovitz, Erica Weiss, Felix Weiss who although have passed on, their legacy of love and appreciation for life and everything good in this world, have and will continue to shine through me for all the days for the rest of my life. My brothers, David, Dany, and Jonathan Horovitz, words can't even begin to describe how unfair it would be to compare you to any other. There are simply no equals and you are perfect. My uncle Michael Friedlieb, you have positively impacted my life more than you'll ever know and no one could ever come close to replacing you in their wildest dreams. Simply put, you have singlehandedly set a new standard and world record for World's Best Uncle. My wife Nelly Horovitz, I'd like to express my deepest gratitude for your love, support, and patience while crafting my thoughts into words throughout this process and beyond. The life we are creating together with our two beautiful children Benjamin and Rachel, while watching them impress us daily, are constant reminders of why living a life filled with love, generosity, and above all, family, are simply the greatest riches.

Contents

Prelude

Promoting Lifelong Wellness

There is no important, underlying purpose for the aging process, and I will never be convinced otherwise. The term 'process' itself, seems premature, doesn't it? As if the path towards our demise is well calculated and governed by certain rules and regulations. Chaos and torment, is more accurate, in my opinion. Ironically, we deteriorate from the very same forces of nature, which are responsible for keeping us alive in the first place.

If Disney's The Lion King, has astutely taught us anything, just because one life ends, does not mean that life itself ceases. It is all part of the great circle of life, isn't it? When animals die, they decompose and simply become part of another aspect of the food chain. Therefore, we should all take comfort in knowing, that everything is ok, because the worms need us as compost. "Ah but that's still life", my colleagues remind me. "Rob, you need to think bigger than just yourself. You need to see the forest for the trees my friend." They continue. "Death is just another part of life; a magnificent journey, if you will. If you could only see how beautiful it truly is," as if they're speaking from experience. Without making this book about spiritual and religious beliefs, I wish I could believe them, I truly do.

I say that we're all plagued but, "perplexed" is an understatement in describing the feedback I receive from people who just simply are not consumed or fearful by aging, as much as I am. I understand that "consumed" is a negative word, which I shouldn't really use in a book dedicated to inspiring others and promoting lifelong wellness. Still, I think about it quite often. In many cases while conversing with close friends and colleagues regarding what I believe to be the single most important medical topic on the planet, I am often met with a look of confusion.

Puzzlement, as to why I'm bringing up such "deep" subject matter. Disconnect, as to why I completely reject the notion that 'it is what it is' and that we should simply accept and move on. I don't pretend to know what others are thinking, however I can tell you that the reaction I receive when discussing the aging process, is often met with verbal suppression. As in, friends often don't even want to get into it. I completely understand why of course. It's a reminder of our mortality and so why bother thinking about that? There is no purpose spending time thinking and discussing a problem, which has no solution, is there? Well, I suppose the perceived solution by many, is simply that aging and death are the natural way of things. Personally, I find the best time to even consider postulating such a radical question, is when I'm lying down, often before bed.

I often wonder if we as a race have given up in taking the aging question seriously. I certainly haven't. The aging question; there's a term for you. Who are we to question aging? Or at least when we question it, do we really believe we can find an answer? Maybe we have gotten used to existing merely generationally. One person lives and is lucky enough to meet their partner, or not, depending on who is reading, they have children who then are lucky enough to have children and so forth. Those who are fortunate enough to live and truly get to know their grandchildren and in fewer cases, great grandchildren, are considered to have lived long lives. Have you ever noticed that when learning about a death in someone's family there are different reactions, depending on how old the deceased was? A short life is often viewed as tragic, but in our culture there seems to be a knee jerk reaction for the death of someone who has lived up until their ripe 90's or later, as being "lucky". I don't disagree, mind you, but only in the context of relativity amongst those who succumbed to earlier, even more tragic deaths.

On top of it all, type of death is also a huge factor. Have you ever thought of someone passing in their sleep as being fortunate in some way? Quick, painless, and peaceful, in comparison to many of the other horrendous ways to go. The truth is, none of the current options are truly good ones, they're just less bad, aren't they? If I had it my way, I wouldn't die, period, would you? I'd want to live as long as I could with as optimal a quality of life as possible, but maybe that's just me.

I agree that someone in their 90's or later, is absolutely lucky to live longer than most. Still, succumbing to the ultimate end, should still warrant a tremendous level of compassion and empathy for them and their family, shouldn't it? Ten, twenty, or even thirty year differences are huge undeniably, as there are many who pass away in their 50's and 60's or earlier. 70 years of age is viewed by many to be getting up there, however the difference between living that long and then living to join the centurion club, is virtually a lifetime. Imagine 30 years of extra life. What would you do in order to be granted that kind of extension on your time here amongst the living? My guess is probably everything and anything. Of course, while life extension depends on many factors, surely quality of life is a major consideration as well. As arguably the most intelligent life in the universe, shouldn't we be investing more in the quest to solve our ultimate demise? I think, yes.

Currently, our best scenario is surviving through our lineages. Don't you think generational survival is a far, far, far next best scenario? If you didn't age, or at least lived for hundreds, if not thousands of years would there even be a need to have children? Never mind need, would you want children (if you currently do)? If you still did for many reasons, would you perhaps not necessarily have them at the same age? Maybe you would choose to have kids much later in life. Does our mortality play a role in why many of us prefer children at a younger age? We want to be youthful parents and capable of interacting and relating to our kids while we still can, right? Everyone is different in their opinion here, but I'm just picking your brain. I hope you don't mind.

A common answer to aging, is population control. "Imagine what we would do if everyone lived forever? It would be catastrophic. We need the aging process to maintain balance". After giving this much thought, I realize what a bunch of nonesense that is. People are afraid, plain and simple, and I am absolutely one of them. This is a ridiculous conversation, isn't it? While giving a lot of thought to this section, I must admit that I am still considering whether I should even be spending time writing about this, but I promise you there is a method to my madness.

I mean after all, why do we take medication, let alone elevated cholesterol seriously, if not as an attempt at improving both quality and quantity of life itself? Although there are many ways in treating disease, attempting to understand how life works and then how life ages, offers a drastically different perspective on treatment options for disease, than that of the reductionistic, short term model, which modern medicine has adapted. That is, digging deep into our biochemistry, searching for that one molecule, and then that one pill, which will explain it all, isn't where I personally think the answer lies. Do you?

I'm proposing, that our precious molecule might very well be right under our nose and we don't even know it, not necessarily as the elixir of life, but rather as a focal point of understanding some of our most important risk factors that we can influence, for improving quality as well as quantity of life. Many of the same factors, which impact cholesterol health itself, affect the way the body functions, in general. Although I don't have access to the fountain of youth, in using a WISE™ approach to maintain healthy cholesterol, I believe that we can gain a better understanding of what it means to truly promote lifelong wellness in the broader sense.

Dr. Rob's WISE™ Approach

W	I	S	E
Whole: nutrient dense foods, mindful of	Inflammation	Stress	Energy (sugar/energy metabolism)

While contemplating writing an anti-aging book originally, I realized the most common causes for human death in developed countries, revolve around inflammation, sugar/energy, and stress. Not only are each of them intimately connected, but they influence health concerns pretty well across the board, including the best of what we know regarding the aging process. According to the World Health Organization, the top two causes of death are heart disease and strokes. Infection follows, notably with respiratory illness taking up a relatively large piece of the pie.[1] Interestingly, virtually any infection is discovered through an inflammatory/immune response, which is of course influenced by both sugar and stress. Well, as complicated of a topic as this is, here goes.

Introduction

The Mother of All Molecules

There have been many promises of unique substances found in nature, to have had incredible drive towards the utopian dream of immortality; the Fountain of Youth. In the end however, they all succumb to the truth, which is that the human body appears too complex. This was the answer given by Dr. David Sinclair of Harvard University, when inquired in a televised, 60 Minutes interview, regarding a substance that he has his team have been investigating; resveratrol (rez-vera-trol) from red wine. [1] While having incredible success in extending lifespan of yeast through caloric restriction, it was discovered that a gene called SIR2, activates the production of proteins called sirtuins (sir-too-ins). [2]

Revered as a "miracle substance" by many, resveratrol was found to activate these proteins in test tube models, warranting further study. [3] In 2006, Dr. Sinclair was part of a research group investigating resveratrol's ability to dramatically increase the lifespan of mice, with noticeable improvements in insulin's ability to work better as well as cellular energy metabolism, and motor function.[4] Just a few years following in 2008, Dr. Sinclair's co-founded company Sirtris, which is leading an effort in this type of research, was acquired by pharmaceutical giant Glaxo Smith Klein for $720M.[5] Is it hubris on our part to always seem to peg our scientific shortfalls on our complexity? Maybe the answer is in fact a simple one, lurking right under our noses. Either way, I'm grateful for what scientists like David Sinclair are pursuing. They are taking this mission head on and focusing on a topic, which most people seem to just want to forget about. In fact, he admits in the interview, that defocusing is in itself hindering our progression in understanding and overcoming the important issue of aging. I completely agree.

Still, when discussing complexity and placing human beings at the top of the food chain, I can't help but think about other life forms, which have much longer lifespans. Sea turtles live hundreds of years. I remember as a kid being in awe as not only were they beautiful creatures, but they had longevity unparalleled within human beings. When I brought focus to this issue, my teachers would respond in saying "yes but look how slow they are". This truly exemplifies to me how far we have yet to come in our understanding of aging. Does it really matter what the animal is physically doing? I mean would it be more impressive if they lived for hundreds of years, but were able to dunk a basketball too? Actually, I suppose that would be more impressive if anything, but you know what I mean.

Trees are pretty complex too. Sure they don't walk around or talk very much, but they change, and are surely exposed to the elements. Trees are at the mercy of nature, yet live so much longer than most other forms of life here on Earth. How is it that a tree can live past one thousand years? Is it simply because their cells and cellular processes within are so much simpler than those of human beings? I just don't buy it, do you? We're talking ten and often more than ten times that of some of our oldest people. From a cellular point of view, in many ways plant cells are compared to that of animals and undergo extremely complex processes such as photosynthesis, allowing them to convert sunlight into energy. This process and many others I imagine are at similar risks of undergoing oxidation and surely stop working as well over the long haul.

Maybe the fact that trees obtain most of their energy from sunlight as opposed to food is where the answer lies. Food most certainly is damaging, yet necessary; a catch twenty-two really. Food undergoes incredible changes, from cooking methods alone. Perhaps it is our minds, which betray us. Maybe food in general is the forbidden fruit. We allow our emotions to dictate what and when we eat, as well as how much. Is it possible that trees take in only that which they need, as opposed to what they want? Complex, isn't it? Certainly, it can't possibly come down to one molecule.

When I was a naturopathic medical student, although academically food knowledge is a strong-suit within the profession, I was originally fascinated by orthomolecular medicine. That is, using high dosages of isolated molecules, already used naturally within the human body, in order to help physiological functions work properly, or at least more efficiently. As a guy who has always loved the sciences, university, biology curriculum, was full of interesting molecules. I don't know why I never thought, that any one of them could simply be isolated, mass manufactured, and sold as dietary supplements to facilitate better overall human health.

In biology, we are taught that glutathione peroxidase (glut-ath-eye-on per-ox-i-daze) is the 'mother of all molecules' for our natural antioxidant defense system in the body. This system is present everywhere, including our brain. In fact, despite a lack of research proving the famous food additive MSG (monosodium glutamate) causing specific illness, reductions in glutathione while increasing the very enzyme which breaks it down (glutathione-s-transferase) have been reported.[6] MSG has also been shown to increase catalase and superoxide dismutase as well as induces lipid peroxidation, which are all proponents of severe oxidative stress, placing tissues at greater susceptibility of damage. Neurotoxicity in the brain, obesity and other metabolic defects, "Chinese restaurant syndrome," and deleterious consequences on sex organs, are some of the additional well noted areas of focus. [7] While studying glutathione as a 'miracle' substance in textbooks, we were simply asked about enzyme pathways and its role in human health, but never did we ever discuss physically taking glutathione as a supplement. I'd like to point out that "Chinese Restaurant Syndrome" is unfair to the Chinese People as North Americans consume copious amounts of MSG within common household snacks such as potato chips, crackers, and processed foods.

Several years later, I discovered that indeed the rest of the human race caught on and the supplement was born. Though there are several different forms, breathing glutathione from a nebulizer (vaporized mist) is more efficacious than orally in pill form. The theory is due to absorption, yielding better overall results. Either way, I found this fascinating. Yet, glutathione wasn't the only natural substance brought to market. It seems nowadays there new 'flavours of the week,' constantly.

I'm not certain where the obsession began, but I have a feeling due credit is owed to Dr. Linus Pauling. He was the man who is credited for bringing much light to high dosages of vitamin C in supplemental form. It was an amazing idea, no question. Vitamin C serves incredible functions in the body, as I'm sure you are already aware. Of notable mention, are associations with decreasing amounts following activation of our stress response. Although no specific link has been established as of yet, promising observations have been made.[8] Adrenocorticotrophic hormone (ACTH) secreted by the pituitary gland, signals the adrenal glands to produce and release cortisol, one of our major stress hormones and vitamin C is thought to play a role. Interestingly, vitamin C has been used therapeutically for decades in the treatment of mental illness.[9,10] Dr. Abram Hoffer's research using megadoses in the treatment of Schizophrenia among other mental illnesses, holds true still today as a large contribution to the medical profession in my opinion.

Vitamin C is involved in collagen production, which in terms of connective tissue health is paramount. This is why it's use in cosmetic creams for skin health, notably wrinkles and anti-aging, is increasingly prevalent in the market place. In fact, a study revealed that when human connective-tissue cells were exposed to vitamin C for prolonged periods of time, collagen synthesis increased eight fold.[11] In terms of hair, skin, and nails, with collagen being one of the major components, vitamin C is truly eye opening. Then again, what about joint health? Collagen certainly has its place among athletes, as well as prevention of joint injury in people with or prone towards developing osteoarthritis.[12] As a potent antioxidant, vitamin C has been studied at very high dosages, in cancer research[13] and even in the realm of anti-aging science.[14]

While at first I was impressed at the research, my perspective has radically changed in the last few years, as isolated substances have become a dime a dozen, and are simply a shadow in the infinite complexity that is the whole from which they were derived. Pycnogenol (Pike-nodge-N-ol) is an incredible molecule as well derived, from the bark of pine. The antioxidant properties are marketed to be unmatched and since a current trend of thought behind disease and aging is oxidation, taking substances that can counter the process, are highly sought after. If we are slowly but surely oxidizing more rapidly than we can prevent, then we may be rusting in a sense. Much as with vitamin C, pycnogenol is implemented in skin care lines and these tend to comprise of the most expensive products on the market. Pycnogenol has been studied in psoriasis, which is an autoimmune condition whereby skin cells tend to replicate more rapidly as a result of excess inflammation. This causes a kind of silver, scaly look to certain areas of the skin, typically over the outside of the knee and elbow, and is itchy like you wouldn't believe.

One of the more common medical treatments for psoriasis along with many inflammatory skin conditions, corticosteroid creams, having their own host of side effects such as thinning of the skin. Dermatologists will likely inform their patient that psoriasis is a lifelong condition, that can be managed but not cured. Pycnogenol exhibits both antioxidant as well as inflammatory modulating properties by having an effect on one of the controlling genes called NF-kappa beta, an interest point in endometriosis-related pain in women and various other health conditions.[15,16] While this is wonderful in many respects, as with most isolated substances, pycnogenol lacks complexity, synergy, and above all, long term safety data.

Hold the phone, there's something new [sarcastic tone]; another advanced discovery called astaxanthin (asta-zan-thin). As with pycnogenol, astaxanthin is an incredibly rare and antioxidant rich pigment found in algae and salmon. As with pycnogenol, vitamin C, and resveratrol, astaxanthin warrants further research in many avenues such as oxidative stress reduction, skin health improvements, inflammation, cognitive performance, and more.[17,18,19,20] Maybe we should isolate and concentrate astaxanthin from its natural sources and sell it as an ultra-premium supplement. Guess what? We did. It worked. At least it worked in terms of a business strategy and sales [more sarcasm]. Skin care and supplement lines, designed with the intention of slowing the aging process and offering antioxidant support, highly leveraged this idea and charge an absolute premium for it. Are you confused as much as I am? With the industry being flooded with new isolated compounds all the time, how do we know which one will give us the biggest bang for our buck? Will the literature shed some light on the matter?

I'll help you out on that one and just let you in on a little secret. The literature can barely agree on anything as there are conflicting studies all the time.

One day a molecule is revered for something positive, and the next, another study suspects possible side effects. Are you familiar with EPA & DHA (Omega-3) supplements? What about super concentrated, super potent EPA or DHA? Although there have been some fabulous studies showing benefit for inflammation and heart disease, taking EPA supplements long term may increase risk for prostate cancer, a recent article eluded.[21] The industry of course came back with all sorts of backlash, suggesting design flaws in the study.[22]

While I happen to agree with the industry here on this one, I suppose my ultimate point is that there are many poorly designed studies within the supplement space and thus more times than not, leave the public with uncertainty. Science itself isn't perfect; it's flawed, big time. However, it is also the continuous pursuit of the truth. How are we supposed to believe that the 'poorly designed' EPA study, is any different than those pertaining to astaxanthin, pycnogenol, vitamin C, or any other unique, isolated substance out there? I suppose the answer is to simply look at every piece of literature and investigate thoroughly, but what are the odds that the average consumer is willing to go to those lengths? I'm guessing not many. There are peer reviews, summarizing large volumes of literature in one, well-articulated, simplified paper. Still, people are confused and I don't blame them.

I'm going to take a wild guess here, but aren't there 'kagillions' (ka-jillions: made up word) of molecules out there? Are we really going to try and uncover every single one in hopes of finding answers to our complexity issue? After all, how complex is one molecule anyway? Then again, I should be careful, as one molecule can be the difference between life and death, quite literally, such as water. Even cholesterol; how about that? What if we decided to remove cholesterol from food, marketing it to people as a nutritional supplement? Would the body use unoxidized, isolated cholesterol, in the same way as from real, whole food? I bet you not.

The idea of orthomolecular medicine is interesting. Molecules, existing in nature and even within the human body, isolated, concentrated, and taken as a drug. However, inherent flaws lie both in safety and efficacy. Astaxanthan is found in salmon. Within the context of whole food, this molecule is incredibly complex and very healthy as far as the scientific community can tell. Whether the same holds true when isolated, I'm not so sure. A colleague of mine described a situation where a coffee mug is smashed to the ground, breaking into hundreds, if not thousands of pieces, and then meticulously glued back together again. She asked me whether it would still work. My answer was yes. She then asked me whether I thought it would work as well.

David Sinclair admits in his 60 Minute's interview, that he almost fell of his chair when he found out that a possible life extending molecule was found in red wine, no less. While having astonishing low rates of coronary heart disease in France, staple diets consist of foods that are rather high in both cholesterol and saturated fat, two large risk factors; The French Paradox, as it's called. [23] Since wine is one of the commonalities, you can imagine the thrill in learning about resveratrol's potential as the elixir of life. Still, his observation about human beings in compared to mice and yeast in terms of complexity, surely is thought provocative. While I'm not really questioning the difference between us and our single celled organism friends (yeast), I can't help but wonder how resveratrol is any more complex than any other incredible find.

It seems as though each great molecular discovery is notable for interacting with one small component of the human genome better in isolation than any other, which have been tested in isolation. So, if SRT2 is a gene that acts to control sirtuins, which are implicated in the aging process,[24] and we have a database of say thousands or more unique compounds, influencing whether or not this gene is turned on or off, the question often becomes, which one will influence sirtuin the most? In this case within certain parameters, it was resveratrol, which just so happens to be in one of humanity's favourite beverages. Since moderate amounts of red wine have been suspected in conferring certain disease protective benefits, imagine how ecstatic researchers were when resveratrol increased the lifespan of both mice and yeast. "Ah ha!" they exclaimed in their glory. "Everybody, drink up. We did it!"

I loved university life even though I never truly experienced it by definition. Living on campus and enjoying the fruits that come along with that perceived right of passage, was never in the cards for me, however I enjoyed simply learning on campus nevertheless. As a kid, my dream was medicine and I knew that university would be a necessary stepping stone, so from the age of 16 onward, I worked part time and saved as much as I could to put myself through school. When Wal-Mart entered the Canadian market in the mid 90's, I was first in line, handing out resumes. In my home town of Newmarket, Ontario. I started in the garden centre and it was an amazing gig for a 16-year-old. Unlike most, I got to spend most of my time outside helping people with their gardening needs. Carrying topsoil for customers was fun as well as an excuse to catch some rays, while engaging in fantastic conversations with people. Plus, in all honesty, at 16 years old, who was I to say no to helping 'women in distress' carry some bags of fertilizer to their cars?

I will never forget the one time I fell asleep on the job. Bodge was one of the best managers that I ever had. He respected hard work and was incredibly fair. He was the guy you just wanted to work hard for, because you knew how much the company meant to him. I was exhausted, as I chose the hardest course load, I could in high school, because I thought it would give me the best chance of getting into science when I graduated. In retrospect, I was accepted, so no complaints.

Still, working 4 days a week while striving for straight A's, is no easy task as many students will admit. In trying to save up as much money as I could, I limited myself to spending twenty dollars per week and tried to work any extra shifts that I could pick up. Actually, when school was out for the summer, I would work 14-16 days straight, take 1-2 days off, and then repeat. I'm not trying to make it seem as though I worked any harder than the average student, I'm merely setting up a point.

After a year of working straight through the school year, followed by working full time during the summer, towards the end of the season, the Garden Centre slowly became dismantled. As fewer customers appeared, I was the only staff member left working. One lonely shift, my eyelids felt heavy like lead and I fell asleep on the job for a few minutes. I awoke only to see my manager standing right in front of me. I was embarrassed and scared out of my mind that I would lose my job. The reason he came over, he admitted, was to inform me that the garden centre was now closed, and offered me to stay on with the company, moving into electronics, which was by the way the absolute coolest place to work in the store. He told me that he appreciated my hard work over the summer, but that if he ever caught me falling asleep again, I'd owe him five dollars to the "HBF"; the Help Bodge Fund. I never did and wherever he is now, I truly hope that he was promoted to a district manager at least, as Wal-Mart is very lucky to have him, should he still work there.

I worked at Wal-Mart for eight years in total and was involved in the building of a store from the ground up with my brother Dany. I met many incredible people from all walks of life there. Some were students like me, others single parents. Several folks immigrated from other countries to start new lives. I met a gentleman who was a chemical engineer from Iran, while working in sporting goods. An extremely intelligent and all around decent human being. He came to Canada to improve his family's lives, and although he was very well educated, his credentials were invalid here in this country. He would have to pretty much start from scratch.

I met people who suffered from a variety of illnesses, from aches and pains to severe heart disease, among others. The person who typically greets you at the door when you walk in, is often someone truly special. I heard that the credential for that job is "life experience". I formed strong relationships with these people as their stories were touching and I learned a lot. One gentleman shared insight into his struggles with diabetes. He was slowly going blind in one eye and his wife had health issues as well. All I could do was lend an ear. These were genuinely good people who were working hard, and appreciated what Wal-Mart had to offer in terms of health benefits and discounts on store items for their families. It was a culture, working there, and the relationships people formed were strong and supportive. My interactions really fortified my intentions of pursuing health care as a profession. More than anyone though, were the elderly who truly influenced me. Stemming from my grandparents of course, but then people I crossed paths with and mere strangers as well.

I used to walk 45 minutes to work or take the bus if it ever came on time. Sometimes the 55C in Newmarket took longer to arrive at the bus stop than if I went by foot. Remember what it was like to wait for the bus before GPS? Today a rider will know exactly when the bus is going to arrive, leaving opportunities for grabbing a coffee or a snack and still be on time. In the freezing, skin cracking cold of the Canadian winter, waiting for 10 minutes felt like fifty, and fifty felt, well, like eons. One day while waiting outside on the bench for a bus, I sat next to an older woman. She looked like she was in her 90's honestly as I recall wondering what she was doing waiting in the cold. We started talking about topics that I can't recall, but nothing related to health.

By the end of the conversation, she looked at me and told me that I was destined for something special. She asked me about what I wanted to do for a living in the future and when I told her medicine she told me that she knew it. I don't know how and I'm still to this day not even truly sure what I said to spark that confidence. In fact, for all I know she said that to all the young men she met at bus stops. Either way I never forgot it and often think back to her when contemplating health and medicine, particularly now while discussing the aging process and how it relates to maintaining healthy cholesterol levels.

By not staying on campus, along with my years working in retail, I was able to pay for my undergraduate degree in full without any debt. I truly loved every minute there as a result, and I'm not saying it's the only way, but it worked for me. It doesn't take much for me to feel as though I'm doing something important, and that in of itself is gratifying, which is how I felt in University. It's actually how I got hooked on coffee in the first place by the way. I began looking forward to morning coffee with my Dad, but after taking three buses and an hour and a half to get to school every day, one appreciates their time spent on campus I think.

I always looked forward to grabbing a fresh, crisp National Post from Student Centre, carrying it under my arm to the cafe. As thousands of people pooled into the university every morning, it was an exciting place to be. With a student body of about fifty thousand, the daily hustle and bustle was inspiring. Carrying that newspaper while standing in line at a campus cafe, waiting for my beverage, felt intelligent somehow. My guilty pleasure was simply sitting down every morning for about thirty to forty minutes or so, prior to class, watching people go by. It's odd, although intuitively carrot cake by name would seem to be the healthiest choice, the shier fat and sugar content make for one incredible indulgence.

A Question of Genetics

There's that one person who always raises their hand in the middle of class to ask something. Perhaps it's hubris, feeling as though their question is important enough to interrupt the precious time of hundreds of other students. To the 'peanut gallery' in the back of the room who come in to complete their time and leave however, its merely a person's infatuation with the sound of their own voice. Was it courage, intrigue, or engagement? Maybe it was just the carrot cake, but at times I admit, I was that guy.

I don't know what prompted me to enrol in the most difficult course load I could muster within the pure and applied science program. Maybe it was a fear of failure. Despite my registration counsellors advising against such a rigorous schedule, I suppose it served as a defence mechanism in case I wasn't accepted into medical school. I had worked so hard and saved up all that money, that graduating simply wasn't enough. Knowledge would bring me a sense of accomplishment which no one could ever take away. As a result, I enjoyed some incredible lectures.

I loved university so much, that transitioning professions from medicine to academics had crossed my mind often. I think interacting with my professors gave me a real kick. The greats were inspiring, and the horrible ones were examples by which to never follow. Such characters, they were. There were better dressed profs, and there were those who were always late no matter what. Some made unsurpassed efforts to get to know their students despite large class sizes of several hundred students, whereas to others, I was merely a number.

As I recall, genetics was a particular treat. The professor was medium in height for a man, say 5'8", and was a stalky fellow, I suspect in his late forties. With sort of a Philip Seymour Hoffman haircut, his medium, long red hair was parted to the side and he was sort of quirky in nature, frequently arriving to class with his briefcase barely holding all of his random papers together. He always waltzed in with a smile and answered any questions we had before beginning, which was counter to how most of his peers worked. Have you ever had a class that was truly dynamic and vibrant where the teacher spoke with you and not at you? He would ensure participation and real time thinking. I often suspected that maybe his lectures were prepared on the spot, but either way I appreciated every minute of it.

He recommended an incredible book by Judith Hooper called Of Moths & Men. This is a fascinating history of university professors attempting to prove evolution visually, using moths in England during the industrial revolution.[25] The description, particularly in the way of character development was enchanting in a way. My genetics prof was clearly one of her characters in my mind. In fact, I wouldn't be surprised if following lecture, he took his notes to a classy pub, sipping on fine brandy, while indulging in his life's work. He never gave us any impression that he was an alcoholic whatsoever, on the contrary, but something about him suggested a type of perceived 1900's academic class. A rarity, indeed.

It was during a cellular repair and mutation lecture, that the wheels began to turn. The human genome project was really an exciting frontier in science as it still is to this day. Genes however are often misrepresented in my mind by people who call themselves experts on the subject, tending to simplify as though we truly understand them, when in fact, we haven't the slightest clue. Discerning exactly what a gene does and how it operates, providing the human body certain with attributes, is a grain of sand in vast desert, where to find a glimpse of water, is but a faint mirage. No one really knows what genes do. Ok, I'll be kind. I suppose we do; genes make proteins.[26]

Genes make proteins, which lead to mind boggling sequence of events, that can change without notice. Imagine the complexity of a country's road system. One road leads to another road, giving more options which each lead to more options, with even more options, and so forth. The road system of an entire country is 'little orphan Annie to Godzilla,' in comparison to the shier magnitude by which a gene signals the creation of a protein. Each protein created or not created by genes (as the case may be), lead to numerous possible outcomes which are all dependant on other numerous outcomes of their own, all which change on a dime, possibly contributing to numerous possible outcomes, we think. Does your head hurt yet? I know mine does.

Genes act as sort of 'on/off switches'; starting points for entire blueprints of physiological responses. Perhaps one of the most complex examples that I can think of at the moment, is inflammation. NF-κB (nuclear factor kappa-light-chain-enhancer of activated B cells) or NF-kappa beta protein complex, is created by several genes and is such a switch, assisting in turn inflammation on when we need it, and off when we don't. As complex of a task this is, the tip of the iceberg is an understatement when trying to convey how incredibly important this one protein is, in contributing to our very existence as we know it. Although many view genes as finite determinants of who will get what disease, we now know that while predispositions certainly exist, genetics can also be influenced by many factors, including lifestyle choices.[27]

Our cells are susceptible to mutation constantly, and I don't mean the "teenage, mutant, ninja" variety. I'm referring to genetic alterations of course, leading to potential health problems. In class we discussed immune dysfunction, accelerated aging, cancer, among others. Although our bodies seem to have incredible protective mechanisms, cells are particularly susceptible to damage during replication and repair.[28] One might immediately wonder what causes such mutations. A somewhat sarcastic answer is, what doesn't? Everything from radiation from the sun to chemical residues or metabolic by-products from our food, to even pollution found in our drinking water from industrial waste, all represent possibly ways in which are cells may become damaged. A crazy thought popped into my head during class one day. I asked whether cuts and bruises, say when kids fall off their bike, would technically increase risk of developing mutations. I know how that sounds, as how often do you ever hear about scrapes causing disease, do you? Never. I've never heard of it. Still, if cells are replicating faster during healing and developing mutations as a result, why aren't risk factors for say accelerating the aging process or developing cancer increased, even by a little? When I inquired further with my professor, his answer surprised me. Technically, in his opinion, our risk would in fact be increased from a cellular standpoint, even though no research to his knowledge had ever investigated the notion. This idea was the beginning of everything for me.

Every so often in biology, there was a topic, that prompted someone to inquire about the aging process. I found it humorous, that in every single instance, the professor answered briefly, but then moved on, informing us that the aging process was not up for discussion in class. Completing the planned curriculum was more important. The funny thing, is that questions regarding aging were the single most important, and by far most interesting aspects of any biological science lecture. After all; why were we all studying biology if not to learn more about the aging process? Biology degrees are by in large designed as a stepping stone for someone pursuing a career in research, with a common goal of helping either in the way of developing treatments or new testing methods for diseases. Therefore, the mission is to help preserve human life for as long as possible, is it not? This is precisely the way I feel with respect to maintaining healthy blood cholesterol levels. In examining this life essential molecule, although we are often reminded of cardiovascular disease, the underlying purpose of is to improve quality and quantity of life. Cardiovascular disease is part of the aging process, whether we want to admit it or not.[29]

Cholesterol is not really the root of cardiovascular disease, but maintaining its good health may in fact be. I'm not referring to the level of cholesterol in the blood, but rather actual health of the cholesterol itself and the arteries which carry it to our cells. Does that make sense? We are beginning to understand that blood cholesterol levels are only as useful as what else is happening within that artery, or what has already happened to the cholesterol from cooking methods or other influence. That said, I completely understand why most of us are fixated on the numbers our doctors retrieve from lab tests. I know my Mom is for sure. She is always conscious of her cholesterol levels and I don't blame her. I mean, there are reasons why these guidelines exist in the first place and why our esteemed medical associations accept them.

Once a person is already assessed for cardiovascular disease risk (smoker, obesity, etc.), their lab values are then put into context for evaluating further. Certain levels of cholesterol absolutely correlate with increase risk of having a heart attack or stroke and should be taken very seriously, but what I'm about to share with you goes way beyond numbers. While not ignoring possible genetic predispositions, unhealthy lifestyle choices cause cholesterol to behave badly in the first place. Cholesterol means more with context.

I propose that cholesterol is more likely to get damaged as we age, but this shouldn't detract us from examining in context as to why. How the aging process damages our cholesterol containing arteries, as well as our immune system, flourishing within our blood stream, is a topic I very much want to share with you in this book. As the body begins to break down, even in its unaltered state, if present in large enough quantities over a long enough duration, cholesterol can dramatically increase risk of heart attacks and strokes, but we all need to realize something more pressing here I think. Even though heart disease is the number one killer in developed countries, its major root causes might not only contribute to the acceleration of aging as we know it, but influence health problems spanning across the board. Inflammation, oxidation, sugar, stress. These are pretty much the common themes existing throughout the health world, no matter what your health goals are, yet our level of understanding is just beginning to envelope.

The human body is made up of trillions of cells. In fact, a recent study estimates that it ranges in the 3.72×10^{13}.[30] The power to the 13 means 10 trillion, by the way. What boggles my mind, is that for a good portion of most of our lives, we each have billions or trillions (as no one knows for sure) of cells having already, collectively divided billions or trillions of times successfully. How old is one at their best, both physically and mentally? To clarify, I'm not referring to the amount of knowledge, accrued over time, although ability to accumulate and recall information might apply. Perhaps 21? For the sake of argument, let's say 21, give or take a few years.

Think about it; billions upon billions of successful divisions by that time in a person's life. Furthermore, consider that there are a multitude of occurrences that can and do go wrong in a person's DNA, from the time of their creation until the legal American drinking age. Our cells are bombarded constantly, yet regardless of the many environmental challenges such as pollution, deleterious foods that we eat and unhealthy beverages we wash them down with, our various stress levels, to just about anything and everything that we do in life; when we are young, our bodies can take it. We all know this, but are we really giving it due consideration? Over the first 21 years or so of a person's life, their cells adapt. I'm sure you can think of certain exceptions such as certain childhood illnesses, however it is more common than not, that despite all of the awesome obstacles standing in our way, the human body is built with time tested, self-correcting machinery. We heal.

\With 100,000's of possible DNA damaging occurrences daily within our cells, they continue to divide over and over again.[31] Those cells that are destined to divide incorrectly or that are damaged, either self-destruct or get repaired extremely efficiently. We have an enormous array of checkpoints so to speak. In order for cells to divide properly there are safety measures in place to make sure that harmful mutations for the most part will be dramatically avoided in future cell lines. Repair mechanism examples include: direct repair, base excision repair, nucleotide excision repair, mismatch repair, and double-strand break repair. These and more, are prominent within our cellular blueprints, ensuring that devastating mutations do not persist. This is precisely why some scientists, instead of asking why we get cancer or age, prefer the more interesting question of 'why don't we?'

Then, all of a sudden after 21 years or so, we begin declining. Differently for everyone, I know, but consider a 30-year-old versus the 21 and you'll anticipate noticeable differences in most people. One example is what I like to call, the 30-year-old 'pudge face'. Simply join me on a potato chip binge, and bear witness to my face 'pudging' up. I'm not afraid to admit it, nor am I the only one. If you're in your 30's, chances are you experience greater weight fluctuations than during your early 20's, don't you? Wrinkles appear as laugh lines, hair begins to thin. Not huge extremes typically, but you or many of your friend and colleagues are getting there, right? Why is that? Doesn't that frustrate you? For about 21 years or so, our bodies defy universal, entropic, disorder so to speak, creating something beautiful, unique, that is alive and well. If you're older than that, hopefully you're one of the lucky ones who is 'aging gracefully' but you'll know that most people have visible signs, despite their best efforts.

The aging process itself, does not really bother me. I truly have come to terms with the fact that we age or become damaged over time, but what really irks me to no end, is the fact that it doesn't have to be this way, and our existence until the ripe age of 21 or so proves it. In fact, our existence in the first place, proves it. Up to a certain point in our lives, our bodies are seemingly unaffected for the most part by any of the external and internal factors that cause damage to the point of visible aging. With billions to trillions of cells dividing billions to trillions of times successfully, you mean to tell me that with time, cells just aren't as good at it anymore? "I'm sorry to inform you that your cells have divided too many times and don't know how to do it properly anymore. They're tired." You're telling me, that finally, after trillions of times of successfully conquering a plethora of environmental challenges, suddenly our cells just don't know how to continue responding in the same exceptional manner? That makes so logical sense to me whatsoever.

To The Ends of Our DNA

I could understand if after one or two successful divisions, something went wrong and we began accumulating damage, but after trillions of successful runs, why all of a sudden the decline in function? Is it all of a sudden? These are questions that truly get me. Recent evidence seems to shed some glimpse as to what happens. The analogy is that of a photocopier. The first copy always looks best, doesn't it? Most of us have seen what happens when we try to print many copies. Eventually, the latter versions no longer appear exactly as the original anymore. Visible differences such as faded ink in certain places or variations in sharpness, become apparent. Similar things happen within cells, if you agree with the telomere theory of aging.

'Telo' is from the Greek word, which means 'end' and in this case, depicts the ends of our chromosome, containing specific proteins, important, we think, for structural stability, gene regulation, cancer, and cellular aging[32] What first caught my attention quite a few years ago, was a study by TA Sciences in New York, where a discovery of what are now known as telomere activators, were isolated from the herb Astragalus membranous, called TA-65. A commercial age-management product by TA Sciences was released in 2007 called PattonProtocol-1.[33] The idea is that as cells age, telomere length shortens, thus the susceptibility of damage, increased. Research suggests this is due primarily to an enzyme type called telomerase. Telomere activators such as TA-65, inhibit telomerase, maintaining length, which is thought to slow down or even reverse aging. Sounds heroic, doesn't it? I certainly thought so, however it is most certainly too early to tell. Look at anyone who has taken telomere activators over the last several years and I can assure you that they have aged visibly just as the rest of us.

While of course I don't have the fountain of youth in my grasp, I wanted to truly provoke you in thinking about aging and longevity along with quality of life. Relatively few are working on finding any real answers and those who are, have many different theories and approaches. As drugs aim to fight disease, the 'one molecule fits all' approach is certainly an interesting one, as we know how powerful they can be in alleviating suffering, particularly in the short term. While many of these interesting molecular finds have merit, they tend to reveal themselves as brief fads rather than time tested results. Perhaps one of the most interesting compound yet to be explored for not only fighting disease, but shedding light into the most important aspects of our eventual demise, aging, is indeed, none other than, cholesterol. I find it fascinating that all or most research on the aging process can link back to maintaining healthy cholesterol in a big way.

Maintaining healthy cholesterol levels is not necessarily anti-aging. I'd like to point out however that the best of what we currently know in terms of keeping cholesterol working at its best, reducing or maintaining low risk for cardiovascular disease, also includes the very best of what we know regarding the aging process as well as many other health condition ranging across the spectrum. It is my belief that the potential damaging effects cholesterol can have on the body, are in fact many of the same factors, which promote the aging process and chronic disease. Imagine our own mechanisms not working properly or at least up to the best standards that most of us have been accustomed to for some period of our lives. Imagine cholesterol serving as a biomarker for aging, both from a prevention as well as assessment standpoint, which we can analyze and improve upon, right in front of our very own eyes. Help cholesterol work optimally and reduce disease risk and mortality rates pretty much across the board? I don't know. My purpose isn't to bring together enormous pieces of data proving it one way or another. After all, "disease risk across the board" is a pretty serious claim, of which I am not proposing here in this book.

This book is meant for everyone who is interested in pursuing lifelong wellness. I believe we are all capable of making specific changes in our lifestyle, not only in the best interest of cholesterol and heart disease, but coincide with the very best of what we currently know in naturopathic medicine, anti-aging medicine, or any other name by which you choose to give it, without ever confusing yourself with natural pills, powder, or potions, though I will most certainly discuss them. It is not only my pleasure, but a lifelong dream to share with you some of the absolute best of what I know. More specifically, using the maintenance of healthy cholesterol, as a focal point for explaining and connecting inflammation, sugar, and stress, with chronic disease and aging. Here's to promoting lifelong wellness.

Sincerely,
Dr. Robert William Horovitz, B.Sc., ND

Chapter 1:

What Most Cholesterol Courses Teach

The best education was never really discussed in class. Of course it's no surprise as the academic system structures curriculum so to create a standard amongst students, which is fine. Still, truly the best curriculum had been left behind for us to wonder about. Instead, our brain power was spent relentlessly on useless, factual memorization and little actual engagement for physical, real world application. I'm referring to both high school and university, at least in my experience. Doesn't it bother anyone else that students spend full days learning most of which they will never use in real life or remember again? I've brought this point up over the years and am always met with dismay, almost as if people are offended by the question in the first place having gone through the same system as I. You will know what I'm referring to if you are old enough to remember studying before the internet.

Some teachers absolutely insisted on using overhead projectors. They took erasable markers and wrote notes while lecturing on these clear plastic sheets, remember? It was absolutely insane and yet there were always a few people who insisted that they loved learning this way. I say, "good for those people.". During lecture, the teacher jot down notes, which appeared on a projector. Students saw the shadow of a hand, with a marker, drawing in real time. Once the end of the sheet was reached, the teacher had no choice but to erase everything similar to a chalkboard, or perhaps, but rarely, if the school had a large enough budget for more plastic sheets, it would be switched up for a new, clear one, and lecture would continue.

In other words, if you missed a key point that was written, you would never have the opportunity to later revisit unless you received notes from someone else in the class. Oh and by the way, this was just merely in the 90's. Therefore, missing a class wasn't exactly in your favour, if you cared about grades. The crazy part, is that teachers always had the opportunity to simply photocopy original notes or at least offer students the opportunity to photocopy them at their own cost. When asked whether this could be done, some teachers were happy to assist, because obviously it meant that students had a greater opportunity to learn and succeed in their class. Others however just responded with, oh and this is great; "If I gave you my notes, there would be no need for you to come to class." To this day, I'm confused and I'll let you simmer on that one for a bit.

In looking back at least for my own good, I would have loved to have had my time respected more by the system. That is; condensed, focused, and applicable information, as opposed to drawn out, diluted curriculum. Perhaps that's the real direction where education is going now that technology is catching up. Students will finally have more choice in what they are learning as well as how and by whom. In the last few years I have had the privilege of truly taking a step back, reflecting on what I have learned amongst my academic studies. What I realize, is that for the most part, the really good material was kind of just left in the dust.

I have always questioned really long, structured lectures within school systems and maintain that depending on learning style, most of the key points can be learned in a much shorter time frames. This isn't about, who's 'smarter than the average bear,' either. For example, in a three-hour lecture, does the prof really need to always go right up until the buzzer? I loved when really good profs not only allotted time for questions but managed to finish ahead of schedule; all, while still providing benefits of the key take home points. High school biology was obsessed with us memorizing complicated, metabolic pathways such as Glycolysis (Gleye-kol-i-sis), Krebs cycle, and the Electron Transport Chain. Below are three charts to give you an overview of what they look like within our cells. These are by no means complete as they are a continuous work in progress.

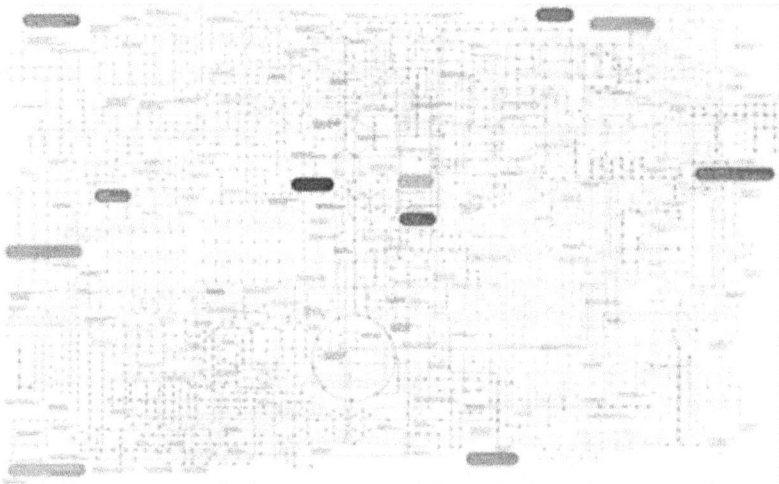

Figure 1(a): Metabolic Pathways[1]

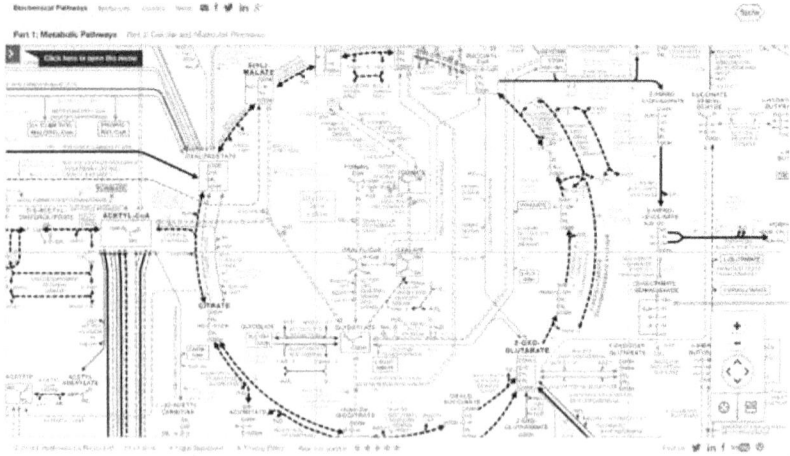

Figure 1(b): Metabolic Pathways[2]

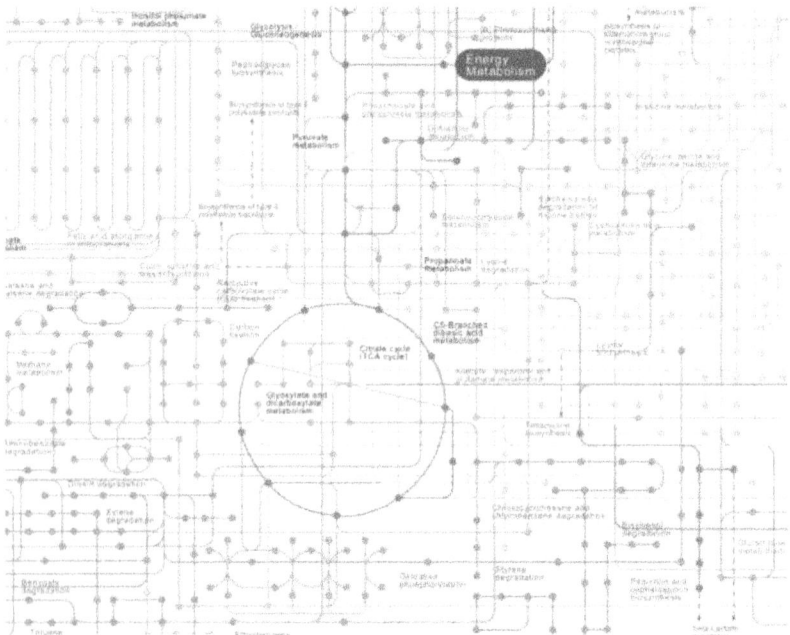

Figure 1(c): Metabolic Pathways

This information is of course meant for research advancement, hardly applicable to undergraduates, let alone high school students. While in university, I thought "surely we're going to better understand how these pathways can positively change lives". Counter intuitively, this was most certainly not so.

No topic has taken a back seat in my view, as much as cholesterol, where lectures almost always start out the same way. I know this because over the years, the topic has appeared numerous times, yet always lacking key discussion opportunities. Lectures typically begin with examining the molecule itself, followed by explaining that without cholesterol, we humans could not exist as a species. Moreover, we aren't the only life forms, dependant on cholesterol. Our fungi neighbours have also evolved with a similar molecule called ergosterol, which they also depend on for survival. In fact I later discovered that anti-fungal medicines such as Imidazole, fluconazole, ketakonazole are predicated on this fact, for a drug which stops ergosterol synthesis, will inevitably stop fungi from replicating or rather compromise their cell membranes[3].

Cholesterol 101

One of the first lessons in biology teaches distinctions between bacteria and plant cells, from animal's. The first two have cell walls whereas the latter does not, and major credit is owed to cholesterol. This versatile molecule assists in creating a membrane around our cells, maintaining semi fluid-like properties.[4] So in other words, our cells are allowed rigidity, but not too much so that they break. Therefore, cells remain flexible and are complex, structurally. Following, text books often share basics regarding cholesterol synthesis such as the fact that most is created in the liver, with a smaller percentage obtained from food, namely animal products such as that tasty slap of velvety, organic, grass fed butter, softening on your kitchen table, only to later glisten on a lightly toasted slice of freshly baked, sourdough bread.

I have had the distinct pleasure of being audience to a multitude of lectures on cholesterol and I have never really given its function a second thought until merely a few years ago. Typically, the flow of information begins at structure, then synthesis, following with physiology. This often touches upon the primary enzyme responsible for cholesterol production, HMG-CoA Reductase. It sounds difficult to pronounce, but if you break it down, you'll be sure to impress. HMG, then Co-A, then Reductase. Now say it fast all together, HMG CoA Reductase.

Since high cholesterol is a pandemic amongst first world nations, cholesterol lowering drugs such as Lipitor and Crestor are what they call "Blockbuster Drugs". Blockbuster, in that they are smash hits, or rather drugs prescribed to an incredibly large amount of people generating over a billion dollars in sales for the manufacturer. [5] These two pharmaceuticals, while belonging to the class known as HMG CoA Reductase inhibitors, do exactly that; inhibit the enzyme responsible for creating cholesterol in our livers (hint: the one you just memorized).

Cholesterol of course is used all over the body. I won't bore you with long details, however here are some keynotes: cholesterol is used to create bile, which is super important in terms of digesting fats as well as helping us to better utilize fat soluble vitamins such as A, D, E, and K. Cholesterol is used by the body to create vitamin D as well as steroid hormones, such as stress and sex hormones.[6,7,8,9] In my experience, quite a bit of emphasis is placed on cholesterol synthesis inside of cells and how it's regulated. Transportation of cholesterol is also an important topic, touching on the different types of cholesterol such as LDL, HDL or 'good and bad', respectively. The reasons of course, is to lead right into cardiovascular disease and some pathology. Finally, the differences between high and low cholesterol are ironed out, and then bada bing, bada boom; a typical cholesterol lecture is pretty much completed.

The amount of studying for a high school student on this topic is pretty advanced relative to most subjects. Memorization of enzymatic pathways and long names such as 'liposomal' and such, are elaborated and tested upon, placing biology tests on the more challenging side. However, when you fall in love with the material, you can most certainly learn just about anything. Moreover, it surely didn't hurt to have an amazing biology teacher in high school; one of the best I've ever had, Ms. Clarke, who I will always credit as one of my greatest inspirations regarding the sciences. She made class fun, engaging, and I'd never dream of taking anything away from what I've learned from her. The curriculum unfortunately, skipped over what I believe to be cholesterol's most pertinent attributes.

Spare Me The University Biology

It was an amazing experience, first year Biology at York University. Bio 1010 housed around 500 students in Curtis Lecture Hall I, a massive auditorium, larger than any other that I've personally seen. Here, students are truly reduced to numbers. I'll never forget, during the first class, the prof asked "how many students are taking this class because they hope to get into medical school?" Almost every hand was raised. Then we were asked, "how many of you believe that those who raised their hands are actually going to get in?" Silence. As the class size shrunk dramatically over the following semesters, a certain truth became increasingly apparent.

Biology as an undergrad really didn't have very much in common with medicine as a practice, but more so was focused on research. Reductionistic, scientific models used to pier deep within our cells, attempting to learn more about their inner workings. Interesting work and unbelievable life's work, don't get me wrong. I acknowledge all of science's deserved accolades. Nevertheless, I recall how disappointed I felt with course material. The mission to improve quantity and quality of life, was never truly entertained. It was as though the curriculum dug so deep inside our precious cells, that it lacked why we were really investigating in the first place.

If someone asked me today what cholesterol is, I would probably contemplate responding with "what isn't it?" or "cholesterol is everything". This is not the real answer of course, as cholesterol is, really a molecule. The Greek translation literally means a bile solid alcohol depending on where you obtain your definition. It's a sterol molecule. The function however of cholesterol is so utterly impressive that I felt inspired enough to write an entire book linking its health with chronic disease and the best of what we know regarding aging. The truth is, most people don't care about its definition, the physiology and synthesis, its rate limiting steps, or transport within the body. I'll tell you what they do care about though; real health concerns. You know; such as stress, menopause, and andropause? In fact, let's start this in reverse.

Chapter 2:

Menopause & Andropause

A ndropause isn't even recognized by the World Health Organization, yet is difficult to diagnosis, regardless. In fact currently, Andropause is viewed by many in the same category as Late Onset Hypogonadism and said only to exist in those men who have loss of testicular function, as a result of accidents, diseases, or following surgical or medical castration due to advanced prostate cancer.[1] Scientists have gone to many lengths in attempting to refine a specific diagnosis strategy but in the end, for most people, the name resonates as part of the aging process in men, it seems. Either way, any woman married to a guy in his 50's or so will absolutely swear up and down that Andropause is real, it exists, and she is willing to volunteer her husband for scientific experimentation just to prove it.

It's like a scene out of a television sitcom. The wife makes an appointment to see a doctor regarding her menopausal symptoms and brings her husband for moral support. The husband is minding his own business, just silently complimenting himself on what a great support system he is, so that he can get in her good books again from all the craziness he's been experiencing with her being in menopause. Little does he know, the appointment was an ambush in the first place, as the during the middle of the visit, the wife says to the doctor; "Wow, you're good doc, you should see my husband for his Andropause. You see honey (looking at her husband), you should book an appointment to see the doctor about your Andropause." The husband thinks, "what is she talking about?" He responds with "What are you talking about? Andropause. I thought we discussed this already. Andropause is a myth. It doesn't exist, right doctor (looking at the doctor)? Please tell my wife it doesn't exist." The doctor looks at her and says "Well, I'm afraid your husband is technically right as it's not a recognized health concern by the World Health Organization." As a result, the wife stops speaking to her husband for a little while and the husband is in a state of utter confusion as to what just happened. No one wins in this scenario.

When a woman reaches Menopause, diagnosis can be made fairly easily after no longer having her menstrual period for approximately 12 months.[2] Additional laboratory analysis often reveals dramatic declines in Estrogen and Progesterone with corresponding symptoms. In men, it's much more difficult to ascertain exactly what happens in Andropause. When looking at the definition, a steady drop in testosterone from the age of even 30 years old is often stated. Irritability, anxiety, low sex drive with erectile dysfunction, and muscle loss, are just some examples which are listed, but ambiguous nevertheless in establishing definitive margins. It is also unclear as to what sort of time span Andropause takes into effect, as in women, from the time their menses stops for the next few years, Menopause is in full force and then disappears. Or does it? We'll expand on this later.

It is not uncommon for men to inquire about their testosterone levels with a doctor and if indeed it is evaluated as being too low, a testosterone deficiency warrants treatment with testosterone therapy. Men are given testosterone to bring their levels back up to normal, in which case they can experience dramatic improvements in their presenting symptoms. It goes without saying however, that these don't come without potential side effects. Excess amounts of testosterone has been linked with increased risk for prostate cancer, but this has been an area of controversy, as there is also a host of more recent evidence arguing against the validity of this 2/3 of a century old suspicion, proposing that the scientific community rethink and re-evaluate this concern.[3,4] That said, testosterone is normally created by the body on a need to need basis and used appropriately. There is a feedback mechanism such that we produce more hormone when is required, and less or none, when we don't, basically. When introducing this sex steroid hormone into the blood stream in the form of a drug, there truly is no telling what will happen with long term use, so careful administration is a must, and even then, the best doctors cannot replicate dosages in the way that the body does in healthy, young men.

Steroids Are Impressive

The bold text within the following definition of a steroid hormone, really stood out in my mind:

"A steroid hormone (abbreviated as sterone)[5] is a steroid that acts as a hormone. Steroid hormones can be grouped into five groups by the receptors to which they bind: glucocorticoids, mineralocorticoids, androgens, estrogens, and progestogens. Vitamin D derivatives are a sixth closely related hormone system with homologous receptors. They have some of the characteristics of true steroids as receptor ligands, but lack the planar fused four ring system of true steroids."

Steroid hormones help control metabolism, inflammation, immune functions, salt and water balance, development of sexual characteristics, and the ability to withstand illness and injury. The term steroid describes both hormones produced by the body and artificially produced medications that duplicate the action for the naturally occurring steroids."[6,7,8]

Basically, steroid hormones do pretty much everything related to the aging process and disease processes themselves, as we know it. That's all, no big deal. I can't help but think, "Hello, did you just hear what you read? Are you listening to yourself?!" Again, I'm just writing out loud here, but shouldn't we be paying just a teeny, tiny bit more attention to these steroid hormones, since they drastically affect our overall ability to function properly? Maybe that's something which shouldn't really be shoved under the rug during lecture, don't you think? We should have spent a considerable amount of time, focusing on just how incredibly important steroid hormones are clinically, before moving on. The gears began turning within this thought train and I thought to myself as I heard the horn, wow, if this locomotive is leaving, I had better get on, fast. 'Beep, beep. All aboard!'

By far, the most interesting thing about cholesterol, is its function in the body. I find it almost comical now looking back that we never really spent much time on what cholesterol can do for us; not really anyway. Instead, we just sort of took that part for granted and focused on clinically manipulating cholesterol in terms of dietary intake highs and lows, assessing cardiovascular disease risk based on our lab values, etc. Even now, seldom do I hear discussion about what cholesterol can be doing in our bodies to help us, when truly that's the entire point of producing and eating it in the first place, I think. It was created to do us good. By nature, cholesterol is designed to pretty much help us with everything humanly important for survival. Let's spend a little bit of time on this concept instead of doing what everyone else seems to be doing, and skim over it like it's just the garnish or an appetizer, when in reality, its indeed the succulent main course.

Cholesterol is a precursor for steroid hormone synthesis, among other things such as bile acids, and vitamin D. The below diagram shows you what some steroid synthesis pathways look like.

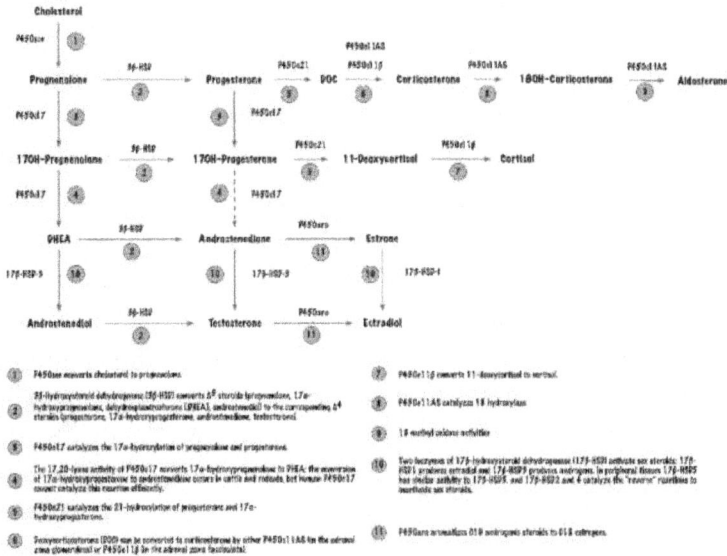

Figure 2: Steroid Hormone Synthesis (recreated from original; Miller, Walter L et al)[9]

A precursor is basically a starting material. In the diagram, notice that cholesterol converts into something, which converts into something else, and something else, and before you know it, boom; estrogen and testosterone. I never really gave much thought to the fact that cholesterol produces steroid hormones as it was simply combed over. Instead, we obsessed over the deleterious effects of cholesterol. What if the real problem is what we're doing to cholesterol and our bodies? It is for this reason, that in addition to managing healthy cholesterol levels, we require a certain level of understanding of what it truly is that cholesterol does.

Hormones, Sports Supplements, and The Fitness Industry

Recognizing that cholesterol is the main ingredient for producing sex steroid hormones, brings all sorts of ideas in terms of how to approach Andropause, Menopause, and Stress Management, among others. However, I'd love to turn our attention briefly to sports medicine. I feel that in looking at health, it's impossible to unlock the best of what we know without looking at athletes as they resemble the best, in many ways what we humans are capable of, physically and probably even mentally. One of the greatest examples in my opinion is bodybuilding. It's a controversial sport. Some bodybuilders themselves even argue as to whether it is a real sport in the first place. These men and women spend years of their lives, decades even, building towards creating their ultimate physiques; truly works of arts. It not only takes incredible dedication both nutritionally as well as physically, but the depth of knowledge, which they leverage every day to self-improve, is truly inspiring.

The question of whether it's a sport surprisingly doesn't even reside in the whole steroid use debate. Not really, anyway. Well, maybe at cocktail parties. The debate is with respect to the competition itself. These athletes, and they are absolutely athletes by the way in every respect, train hard all year to reach new personal heights in hopefully achieving a better version of themselves than the previous year, all to pose on stage on one specific day, for merely a few minutes at best. As complicated as the human body is, here you will see some people weighing in at 200-300 pounds, showcasing incredibly conditioned, lean, ripped muscle. I was intrigued to learn that virtually anything can change the composition and the look of the muscle when it comes to achieving not only a desired physique, but more so one for a very specific period of time. Water content, sodium, food eaten   or not the night before. You name it; many variables need to be considered as a bodybuilder's look may not be at their best right at the time of competition.

There is a plethora of reasons why a bodybuilder may actually look better a week before, or even after the actual day of the show, they are competing for to win. This of course is contrary to most other sports like basketball or soccer where the team either scores or doesn't. If there is only a minute left until the buzzer rings, one team can still win the game as we've seen numerous times. In bodybuilding, that absolutely can't happen. Besides moral support, these athletes are not able to rely on teammates for help while posing on stage for any additional points towards a possible win. What you see is what you get, right there for only a few minutes.

I find sports nutrition fascinating, particularly with respect to how supplements are formulated and marketed towards these athletes. Different sports may leverage different ingredients as that probably goes without saying, but I'd like to use bodybuilders as an example. If you want to lose weight, look to the people in the world that are the absolute best at it. Bodybuilders are probably where the buck stops. I should clarify; bodybuilders are the absolute, undisputed experts in their uncanny ability to both burn fat and build lean muscle mass at the same time. Muscle uses energy to contract, and fat is a source of energy. The leaner muscle that a person has, and the more a person uses their muscles, the better their ability to burn fat. Though many of us rather sit around eating donuts while drinking coffee, hoping for the same results, this is something we all inherently know. Now, not everyone wants to be a competitive bodybuilder, no question. Still, we can scale down from their success, in order to improve our own fitness level and hopefully all around wellbeing.

It's difficult to pinpoint exactly what strategies these athletes are implementing to achieve such outstanding results. Is it because of certain drugs they are taking, such as steroids? Some claim to achieve their physiques by eating a 'Pop-Tarts®

and meat' diet. With intense training and various drug interventions, nutrition doesn't really matter all that much so long as they maintain their macro nutrient requirements. Simply put, a carb is a carb and a protein is a protein, no matter where you get it from. Whether they obtain them from brown rice or Fruity Pebbles, it really doesn't matter, in their opinion.

I don't flat out disagree with this approach from a results perspective, mind you. It's undeniable that there are certain people, whom if they train this way, will absolutely still lose weight and build muscle very effectively. In fact, for the sake of just putting it out there, I had a nutrition professor who outwardly taught the class that technically speaking, if a person enjoys a brisk 20 minute non-stop walk every single day, say brisk enough to break a sweat by the end of it (not 'window shopping' walking), the walk and restricted daily calories to let's say approximately 1500kcal for women and 2000kcal for men, in many cases, it doesn't matter where the calories come from. A person can be eating burgers and fries, yet as long as they adhere to those guidelines, it is likely that they will actually lose weight. The reason can be explained through simple math, which many healthcare professionals use when explaining healthy weight loss to their patients.

If a person walks for 20 minutes briskly every single day, men will burn approximately 3000 calories and women will burn approximately 2500 calories by the end of a day. This is because we are all burning calories even just to stay alive in the first place. Getting up in the morning and brushing your teeth, me writing this chapter, all burn calories. Digestion actually burns more calories than you might think, which is why eating frequent small meals throughout the day may be beneficial for fat metabolism versus fewer large meals; not to mention, ease of digestion. Now, if a man eats 2000 calories and a woman 1500kcal, then how many excess calories are they still burning by the end of the day? The answer is 1000 calories each, does that make sense?

$$\frac{3000 \text{ kcal}}{(\text{men eating})} - \frac{2000 \text{ kcal}}{(\text{men burning})} = \frac{1000 \text{ kcal}}{\text{burning excess}}$$

$$\frac{2500 \text{ kcal}}{(\text{women eating})} - \frac{1500 \text{ kcal}}{(\text{women burning})} = \frac{1000 \text{ kcal}}{\text{burning excess}}$$

Then the question becomes, how many calories are in one pound of fat? The answer: 3500kcal per pound of fat.

In this strategy, if a person is burning an excess of 1000 calories every single day, then by the end of a week, 7000kcal, translating into 2 pounds of fat. This is the reason why most practitioners will suggest 2 pounds of weight loss per week is a healthy guideline for the average person who isn't exercising vigorously and who doesn't have a relatively large amount of muscle mass to begin with. Simple, right? Calories in versus calories out. Or is it? In reality, many factors are at play. For instance, athletes with more lean muscle mass may have faster metabolisms than those with less. Plus, there are other ways of 'boosting' metabolism such as increasing cardio (aerobic exercise: biking, swimming, running, circuit training, etc.), meal amounts and frequency as we've discussed, some supplements very marginally, and nutrient density from food, which I happen to believe is truly undervalued, yet extremely important.

As far as cholesterol and heart disease is concerned, healthy weight loss or maintaining a healthy level of body fat, is one of the most important factors in reducing risk of a heart attack or stroke. Major reasons include; inflammation, oxidative stress, and hormonal health. Seeking professional guidance who can customize a program which best fits where you are at in terms of goals and fitness level, is highly recommended. If you aren't sure where you stand, you may want to consult with a physician before exerting yourself, as not to cause yourself harm. The caloric math above is not meant as a recommendation by any means, but rather for discussion purposes only.

When exercising with weights, it's important to determine what your goals are. Are you trying to lift weights or build muscle? This is a question, discussed often amongst bodybuilders. Strategies for building muscle certainly involves heavy weight, yet the goal is not solely to lift. After all; weights are merely tools in order to help muscles contract. Two main trains of thought exist. The first involves using heavy weights to create micro tears within the muscle tissue, only to respond by creating new fibres. It is this repairing mechanism that creates new muscle tissue. Consistency over a long period of time will result in gaining muscle mass. That said, using extremely heavy weights in order to accomplish mass, is not the only way.

It turns out, that while gradually and safely increasing weight does in fact help to grow muscle, many professional bodybuilders, especially as some of them have become a little bit older and wiser, have begun to think more about the burden of heavy weights on their joints, tendons, and ligaments. This is particularly important if one's goal is to stay as flexible and limber for as long as possible. After all; what good is developing rock hard muscle mass if you lose functionality in the process, right? Therefore, another strategy is to focus on "the pump".

The first time I ever heard the term "the pump" was while watching a very famous bodybuilding documentary called Pumping Iron, [10] starring Arnold Schwarzenegger. Arnold, being at the top of his bodybuilding career while filming, shares with the audience in the movie, a little bit about what the pump entails, which is contracting a muscle in order to literally pump higher blood volumes into the muscle. The muscle then begins to sort of inflate. It pumps up. The theory is that by continuously pumping up the muscle, increased blood is forced in, enhancing nutrient uptake. This not only speeds up healing of any potential tears, but also signals hypertrophy via hormones such as testosterone and growth hormone, naturally.[11]

You don't have to lift heavy weights in order to get a really good pump, as it turns out. Rich Piana, professional bodybuilder and owner of 5% Nutrition, has long maintained that bodybuilders distinguish themselves from weight lifters, as that would imply lifting weight. He mentioned in a recent 2014 interview that high volume, high repetitions, while focusing on contracting and squeezing the muscle to achieve a "burning" pump, is where he has seen some of the greatest gains; both in muscle size and shape quality.[12] A great pump is accomplished by performing an exercise correctly and by establishing what is referred to as the Mind Muscle Connection. Going through a motion in order to move weight may be important for true weight or power lifters, but not necessarily in bodybuilding.

Many athletes insist that it is not the size of the weight that counts. Instead, concentrating on a particular muscle, contracting and squeezing, is the way to achieving a great pump. The amount weight used, is merely a tool used to help facilitate. The side benefit of great form and concentration in this way, is to lower risk of injury as well as accomplish fantastic mass gains. Although I'm not a bodybuilder by any means, rather passionate about fitness, I hold a high level if admiration for what they are able to accomplish.

Supplements tend to over complicate everything. Since physical activity is a great way to improve overall metabolic function and reduce risk of cardiovascular disease, I am often asked which supplements add the most value for someone who is trying to lose weight and gain muscle. My answer almost always revolves around those ingredients which will assist with what more than moderate exercise is designed to accomplish. For example, breaking the body down and repairing can be supported through nutrition and some supplements can certainly be of assistance such as the more famous, L-

Glutamine and Creatine. For the most part however, when listening to most top bodybuilders, whole food is by far the way to go. Athletes are vigilant with their food intake and training for years, achieving stellar results, and only then might they receive some sort of sponsorship by a nutraceutical company.

In reality, many of these athletes never took the supplements which they are promoting. They are getting paid just like any other celebrity does in order to endorse a product. Does that mean these products are bad? No, they can certainly add value; an edge at times. Personally, I'm not a fan of taking isolated caffeine monohydrate, which can be found in many over the counter pre-workout formulas. Can it add value in some instances? Absolutely; energy, motivation, focus, and mild boost in metabolic functioning, certainly provide some shining examples. Still, the best way to burn fat and create muscle is by emulating what bodybuilders do in terms of their nutritional regiment and style of incorporating weights as tools with the right creative intention and form. Real results are earned from consistent, hard work and dedication over time, along with real, whole food. Plain and simple.

Supplements can be confusing to say the least and I don't blame people for questioning what they are taking in the first place. Researching before taking something rather than relying on someone else's opinion is the way to go, regardless of credentials; professional athletes and doctors included. At the end of the day, it is you and you alone who must reap the benefits or consequences of your actions. This in particular holds true in situations where 'flavours of the week,' fad weight loss pills, and false 'cures' alike, seem to dominate and plummet constantly in the media's eye. The truth behind the natural health world as far as building muscle and losing weight is concerned, and as far as reducing cardiovascular risk and truly disease risk across the board for that matter, is what we already know in our hearts. Why must we complicate things? The best medicine that we have ever, and currently know, with all of our research and ambition, has always been and currently is, real, whole, scrumptious, delicious, nutritious, 'food, glorious food'.

I spent years evaluating which sports supplements I thought were the absolute best for supporting my workouts. I have specifically focused on supplements, designed for promoting energy, stress, muscle pump, recovery and inflammation. I began noticing a really interesting pattern. Formulators seem to be fixated on biochemical pathways. For good reasons, mind you, but I'll elaborate further. If you want a fantastic pump while working out, wouldn't it be fantastic if you could take a supplement before you head over to the gym, helping you to reach a better, more sustained pump, using your own body's natural mechanisms? L- Arginine was and actually still is, a very promising such supplement, but there were twists to come. L-Arginine is an amino acid found in various protein sources, naturally. In isolated form, typically at dosages of about 2000mg or so, this amino acid has been placed in many sports pre-workout formulas.

L-arginine can lead to nitric oxide production, causing blood vessels to dilate, allowing for more blood flow. This is a very attractive trait if you are looking for a good muscle pump via increased blood to the muscle, wouldn't you agree? When reviewing an arginine synthesis diagram, it becomes intuitively clear that this substance is a great choice. I'm speaking only of the diagram, not of safety or scientific research at all. L-arginine became revered in the bodybuilding supplement world, yet the push for more intriguing compounds brought about a different perspective on the pathway.

Agmatine, which is in the diagram as well, can also help control the direction of nitric oxide production by acting synergistically with an enzyme called nitric oxide synthase.[13] Without understanding the ins and outs, if you're someone who desires a pump while leaning on supplements to give you as much of an edge as possible, which compound would you choose; arginine or agmatine? Maybe both? Beta-Alanine, another compound, has been shown to increase levels of carnosine in muscles and decrease fatigue in athletes. [14, 15] Maybe you would add in a little bit of that too. Confused? I'm actually not going to argue for, or against any of these options because they all have merit. Still, make no mistake, these items are chemicals, drugs, lacking complexity. They are far from food.

Stop the madness, I say! This type of reductionistic, "pathway logic" is plastered everywhere within the supplement world, ultimately confusing everyday consumers. Plus, results are never really seen through this type of science anyway. Don't get me wrong, they might give athletes an edge but that's the extent of it. Not to mention, the jury is out, regarding safety as there often isn't enough research, particularly regarding long term use. If we really want to get excited about pathways, yielding massive results, it's almost impossible not to acknowledge and spend more time on the one molecule that doesn't receive nearly as much functional credit as it deserves. That 'miracle' molecule, is none other than, cholesterol.

The Mother of Hormones

Menopause, Andropause, and stress are often viewed from the standpoint of pathways, yet the functional aspects of cholesterol always seem to take a back seat, as I've witnessed numerous times now. Allow me to explain. Since testosterone is lowered as men age, increasing its production or at least preventing as much of a decline, is highly sought after. Sure, there are hormone-free herbs such as Tribulus Terrestris, which have been shown as recently as 2013 to increase testosterone as well as act as an aphrodisiac, at least in animal models. [16] However, claims of 'hormone boosting' are rampant within the herbal and supplement world. As a result, scepticism persists in terms of public confidence as to the quality of these products, both in terms of safety and efficacy.

A friend and colleague of mine is passionate about building muscle at all cost, having no fear when it comes to taking nutritional supplements. He will take anything and everything under the sun if there is the slightest chance for the tiniest bit of self-improvement. One day, he called me up with the latest and greatest research on a compound called Pregnenalone, (preg-nen-alone). "Really interesting," I told him, "but I'm not surprised". When he asked me why, I broke down the following diagram for him.

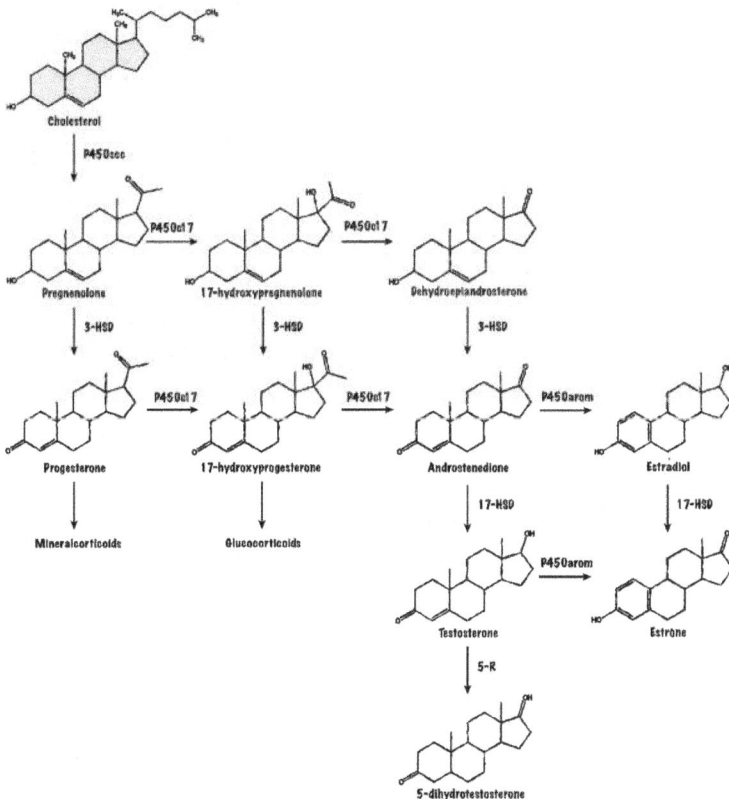

Figure 3: Steroid Hormone Biosynthesis (recreated from original; Janer-Gual G)[17]

Pregnenalone is a precursor for testosterone. In layman terms, it arrives before testosterone in the diagram. Take pregnenalone as a supplement, and according to the diagram, you will increase testosterone production. Sounds romantic, doesn't it? In reality, no one knows for sure whether taking a compound orally in this way will have a reproducible effect that is as simple as what is illustrated. Just because our body can use pregnenalone to create testosterone, doesn't mean that after consuming boat loads, will your body automatically soak it up and think "Ah ha! Just what the doctor ordered!", igniting the testosterone 'rockets' into orbit.

I can't really argue whether taking pregnenalone will or won't in fact accomplish what my friend sets out to. What I do know, is this however; there is no telling what pregnenalone will do, which is the point I really want to drive home. What are the potential side effects of putting an isolated chemical in the body? How well has it been tested? Do we eat pregnenalone? I think you know where I'm going with this. To paint a rainbow after the storm, have another look at the diagram and you'll see something before testosterone and then before that (androstenedione and dehydroepiandrosterone (a.k.a DHEA). While DHEA has been banned from over the counter sales in Canada but available in the US for a few years now, it is marketed nevertheless as a hormone that naturally decreases with age as with testosterone. DHEA is involved in both estrogen and testosterone synthesis as well. For that reason, companies raved about the potential uses as an anti-stress and anti-aging supplement. In reality although there is evidence to support its use, there is also visa versa. I'm hoping that you see the pattern I'm trying to make here. It's almost a giant game of cat and mouse, isn't it? We seem to be searching for specific molecules within a pathway, which lead to what we think is the most desired molecule of them all, for a specific health concern/goal.

Do me a favour and have another look at the diagram where DHEA appears. Notice pregnenalone, and then going back further if you haven't already, you may notice the real tear jerker. Yup, that's right. It's none other than one of the most useful molecules naturally produced by the human body and is widely available in the foods that we eat; cholesterol. The mother load of precursors for pregnenalone and DHEA, and then for both Testosterone and Estrogen, as well as cortisol for stress (glucocorticoids as listed). Of course we wouldn't dream of marketing a bottle of pure, unadulterated, third party tested, super potent, high absorbing cholesterol, would we? Why that would be absolute insanity, wouldn't it? Or is it? I'm not suggesting that you and I should start our own cholesterol supplement company, but I propose that we need to rethink how to apply these pathways in terms of therapeutics.

We create isolated, pharmaceutical grade, pregnenalone, agmatine, and L-arginine supplements and market these chemicals for various claims, despite knowing very little about their safety and efficacy. Yet, we wouldn't dream of ever promoting the use of cholesterol as a healing, natural substance, abundant in the food supply, because that would be considered as extremely dangerous, wouldn't it? Oh, and by the way, it probably would be and I'm in no way advocating the consumption of copious amounts of cholesterol. However, it baffles me as to why we comb over cholesterol in terms of its health promoting ability as though it was some sort of afterthought, while putting our energy into 'flavours of the week' molecules. This type of thinking is absolutely beyond me.

I'm remembering back a past cholesterol lecture. "Cholesterol does some incredible things in the body. It's responsible for creating steroid hormones including estrogen and testosterone," begins the teacher. "Wait a minute." I exclaim. "You're telling me, that cholesterol is responsible for creating testosterone, estrogen, our primary stress hormones, and is probably one of the single most important molecule in the human body?" The professor looks around (I'm making this up by the way) and nonchalantly responds with "Absolutely. You could say that it's the mother of hormones. I wish we could spend more time here, but unfortunately, we have to move on. Just a reminder class; if you can please save the questions until the end as we have a lot to cover today." This is pretty much exactly what happened in virtually every one of the cholesterol lectures I attended.

Chapter 3:

Bone Loss is Worse Than Menopause

Menopause is very easy to diagnose, unlike Andropause in men. Both can hit hard, but menopause is more telling, outright. I don't want to say that women have an advantage, for fear of being clobbered for even thinking of such a concept. However, signs and symptoms are at the very least our bodies letting us know that something is wrong. I suppose that we don't really require hot flashes and depression to accomplish this, when even just visible signs of aging would do. Still, from a diagnostic point of view and to truly distinguish Menopause and Andropause from other health concerns, specific criteria need to be established, and for Andropause it's more difficult.

If you've ever experienced or know anyone who is currently experiencing Menopause, you will know how horrific it is. Some people within the naturopathic medical community have actually called me out on this, saying "Rob, you really need to see the beauty in things. Menopause is part of life. It's truly a beautiful time in a woman's journey, which she really needs to take in, embrace, and to be proud of." Then if I'm really lucky, they'll continue in saying something like "Rob, you mustn't (I'm making the "mustn't" part up) take a woman's femininity away from her". That's when I know I'm in real trouble. Oh, and yes, some people actually speak that way. Menopause is horrible. Period. If every woman on the face of the earth could avoid it completely by having their bodies work the same way that they worked when they were 25 years old, how many of them do you think would say "You know what Rob? Naw, I'm good. Why don't you let all the other women have that magic potion? I'm fine with my hot flashes as it's part of the beauty of being a woman." Yah. That's right. I thought so.

Hot flashes sound quick and painless, like "be back in a flash", but they feel like mini marathons, let me tell you. Or rather, let a woman experiencing them tell you. Mood disturbances is an understatement. A disturbance is like a fly buzzing around you while you're enjoying a good cuppa Joe. Anxiety and Depression from hormonal imbalances in menopause, is a freight train smashing through your living room, during a tornado blast, while someone decided to leave the sink faucet running just for fun. The crazy part, is that even though it's incredibly common and 'normal,' we are not even sure what is really responsible for these symptoms. At first, lower estrogen was suspected as the problem.

Naturopathic Doctors and Master Herbalists alike, may use plant medicines with estrogen-like compounds called phytoestrogens (phyto from plants), which sort of look like estrogen but aren't.[1] They can almost fool the body to an extent and help mimic some attributes of the hormone. This is especially useful in the case where estrogen decreases as in Menopause. Black Cohosh, a herb that has been recommended as a natural menopause remedy for over 30 years, has been thought of as such as herb, though more recent evidence questions whether it indeed does affect the way estrogen is being used.[2] To add fuel to the menopause hot flash fire, decreases in estrogen often result in a relative excess of another hormone called progesterone. One fascinating herb called Chaste-tree has been researched in its ability to affect the downstream production of both estrogen and progesterone, through stimulation of follicular stimulating hormone and luteinizing hormone.[3] Many common menopause herbal formulas found in health food stores these days, contain both estrogenic and progesterogenic ingredients. Eastern, Chinese Medicine has been practicing the use of herbs this way for thousands of years, paying incredibly close attention to balance. Yin and Yang. While in Western Medicine, we often seem to jump on something if we see slight symptomatic benefit, Eastern methods appear to be much more patient and time tested, which has an advantage in many cases with respect to efficacy but even more so regarding safety.

Estrogen is a protector against too much inflammation in the body, and when it drops as in the case of menopause, the health consequences can be devastating. Vascular inflammation for instance, is now gaining recognition in early signs of hot flashes, which certainly brings up the question of concomitant cardiovascular disease risk.[4,5] One of the hardest things I've ever had to say to a woman right to her face was "look I understand that these symptoms are torture." Every time I've said this, and I admit I've said it on more than one occasion, I receive the 'who do you think you are?' look. The 'when was the last time you've had a hot flash, young man?' stare, continued with 'what do you know about torture? You wanna see torture? I'll show you torture!' I sort of take a gulp and dig myself deeper with "but eventually you'll get over these symptoms". I know how that sounds.

Eventually, the common symptoms of menopause will disappear as it only (and I don't use that word loosely) typically lasts for a few years. I propose that perhaps the gravest challenge of all, dare I say more than suffering with tortuous, menopausal symptoms, is the aftermath. Much as a one of a kind, beautiful, cultural, and historical city can be utterly decimated from the tragedies of war, with her foundations crumbling, yielding a mere shadow of what she once was, so too can Menopause exert such a wrath. Essentially, it comes down to estrogen's protective effects against too much inflammation.

Once this hormone drops and inflammation runs out of control, I hate to say it, but hot flashes and mood disturbances make The Big Bad Wolf look like Disney's Ariel, The Little Mermaid. Inflammation is the leading cause of bone loss (vis-a-vis Osteoporosis) and even most of the non-inflammatory causes, are still at least related to inflammation in some way. You may notice that post-menopausal women are at extremely high risk for developing this potentially debilitating disease. However, there are many examples of pre-menopausal women being at high risk for example, such as in the case of lupus, a systemic inflammatory auto-immune disease.[6] Men too are at high risk, and whether Andropause is a real diagnosis or not, testosterone also protects against inflammation.[7,8] Interestingly enough, there are conflicting studies as to whether testosterone is an effective marker for risk assessment or estrogen, even in men.[9]

Symptoms of menopause will eventually end and women will get over it; with the utmost appreciation and empathy regarding just how difficult it is to experience them. Still, while hot flashes and mood disturbances come and go, once bone loss is experienced it's here to stay. Don't let anyone fool you. Can you regain bone density? Absolutely. In fact, there are several successful naturopathic interventions, but require a lot of work, and more than anything, time. To give you an example, it takes approximately one full year before someone will see marginal gains in their bone density, via a DEXA scan. While I don't have the cure for bone loss, the best offence here is a defense. In other words, prevention is imperative. Achieving a better overall functioning inflammatory response is therefore not only imperative for maintenance of healthy cholesterol but rather for minimizing bone loss as well. I will share with you some of my best approaches that I know, right here in this book.

The last point that I really want to drive home with respect to both menopause and andropause is that just because production of estrogen in a woman's ovaries and testosterone in a man's testes drop at a certain point in their lives, doesn't mean that these hormones are lost forever. We know how protective these naturally occurring hormones are, against the real risk factors of bone loss and cardiovascular disease; inflammation. The adrenal glands are typically mentioned when referring to stress, as they produce stress hormones, most famously cortisol and adrenaline. However, that's not all they produce. Most people are unaware that despite age related decreases in Estrogen and Testosterone from the ovaries and testicles, respectively, these hormones are still being produced, using cholesterol in the adrenal glands, located just above our kidneys. [10] Hopefully, you can begin seeing a link between stress, inflammation, and hormonal health, in this way. Maintaining good overall health of our stress response is certainly something not to overlook. I find it interesting that while cholesterol is used to produce estrogen and testosterone, once they drop off, resulting inflammation negatively influences the very precursor from which they originated from. By addressing the fundamentals of what we think causes cholesterol to behave badly in the first place, we can then begin to understand and help cholesterol function optimally so that it can play its role in some of our most important bodily functions.

They say, stress is pro-inflammatory, which is often accompanied with a negative connotation. [11] In truth however, stress and inflammation are both good and bad. Therefore, I'll rephrase what 'they' say as the following: stress can be pro-inflammatory. Here, allow me to provide you with some context. I'm sure you can think of good stressors such as a challenging hobby for instance. With a love of crafting that perfect cup of coffee in the morning, the frustration that can arise should any one variable misfire, is often stressful. Still, it's a passion; a labour of love. 'Good stress.' Since distinguishing between these two forms of stress, having professional interpretation of adrenal function, may be of use.

It's kind of funny thinking about stress in terms of hormones, as we often depict personality traits instead. Maybe it's someone with a low fuse, ready to explode. Then again, perhaps it's that anxious, jittery, worrywart. You may know very well, the person who has been stressed out for so long that they just don't have any gas left in their tank; who barely reacts and is flat out exhausted. None of us want to feel stressed, but our bodies must be at least capable. Our resources and senses such as blood, and sight and smell respectively, must be adaptable. The way we accomplish this, is in a large way owed to hormones. Hormones that are created by none other than, cholesterol.

Some lab tests are better than others at determining where a person's hormone levels are at in terms of normal functioning patterns. Much as clues are to a detective, lab reports shed some light but don't often reveal the whole story. Random blood tests for example, offer snapshots of what certain hormones are doing at the particular moment they are drawn. Therefore, in the case of stress hormone, I tend to gravitate in general towards salivary cortisol panels instead. That is, patients spit into tubes, several times per day, allowing results to be plotted against a curve. This offers naturopathic doctors a fuller perspective of how certain hormones may be behaving throughout an entire day.

Cortisol is one of our major stress hormones, in addition to adrenaline and noradrenaline, both of which are produced in the adrenal glands from cholesterol.[12,13] Without cortisol, we would have a very difficult time managing stress. Not to mention, it serves as a protective mechanism against too much inflammation. As it turns out, Cortisol is by far one of the most anti-inflammatory hormones that we produce naturally in the body. In fact, if you have ever seen a doctor for anything inflammation related, not treated simply by over the counter NSAID drugs such as Advil or Aspirin, chances are, you were prescribed corticosteroids. Dermatologists, use steroid creams as one of their main tools for psoriasis, eczema, and contact dermatitis. Auto-immune conditions involving the immune system attacking itself, also rely on medications such as Prednizone for say the treatment of Crohns Disease or Ulcerative Colitis, among others, which is a corticosteroid.

Perhaps you're an early morning riser who generally feels well rested right off the bat. Conversely, perhaps you're a 'rusty nail' first thing, but once you have your morning Holiday Blend at Starbucks, the gears begin to slowly turn. Then again, maybe your energy peaks later in the evening. In that case, how's your sleep? If you have trouble sleeping, is your problem falling or staying asleep? Do you wake up at night? How many times? These are some of the questions that interest me with respect to stress, as timing of day and relation to sleep is very important for a few reasons.

Adrenal Function

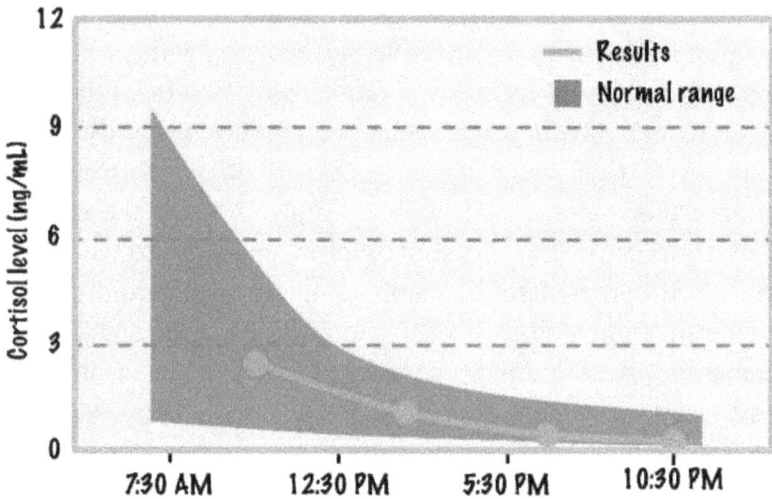

Figure 4: Adrenal Cortisol Curve (recreated from original; Rocky Mountain Analytical)[14]

There's an inverse relationship between stress and sleep, illustrated in the diagram above. Being able to see how cortisol behaves throughout the day not only give you a number of clues as to what's happening with your stress response, but might shed some light on why you may be having those sleep disturbances, helping to dictate the course of treatment, accordingly. After all; prescribing sleep meds seldom offers much to help if anxiety or stress dysfunction is at the root cause. Certainly, medications and herbs alike have their place in alleviating suffering, as there is no substitute for a good night's rest. That said, they are by no means, long term solutions. Here is how cortisol should work.

Cortisol is supposed to be highest in the morning and lowest in the evening.[15] That's not surprising either since you should be at your best performance level right off the bat, following a restful sleep. Then, gradually as the day progresses, stress levels should come down and the body should be getting into relaxed mode so that by the time evening hits, cortisol should be at its lowest, relaxation at its highest, and a person should be able to fall asleep properly, while remaining NeverNeverland until morning. Therefore, when we examine our sleep hormone, melatonin, we should observe the opposite. Melatonin should be lowest in the morning as we should be 'up and atem' ready to seize the day. Then, as evening comes to pass, melatonin should increase. Your own cortisol and melatonin curve can be generated through a simple four-point salivary adrenal gland panel with your naturopathic doctor. No blood, no pain; simple. Although no test is perfect, I hope this offers you value.

Chapter 4:

Feeling Worse as The Day Goes On

As a father of two small children, my wife and I both have an incredible appreciation for good quality, uninterrupted sleep. I admit that I have it easy in comparison to my wife, as at the time of writing this, she is breast feeding my daughter, Rachel, which is not for the faint of hearts. Although gradually becoming easier as frequency goes down and sleep times increase for the little ones, while living through it and other more experienced parents admit that they miss 'those days', it becomes incredibly hard to relate. That's the nice way of saying it, let me tell you. With my son being two years old now, we had the distinct pleasure of deciding whether or not to enrol him in daycare following my wife's maternity leave at the one-year mark. If you've had to go through this decision making process, it's not easy to say the least.

To be honest, I really don't like the idea of someone else 'raising' my kids. I will always insist that the ultimate situation is for my kids to be raised at home by at least one parent. My wife on the other hand, being a workaholic, admits that she would go crazy being a full time Mom and I don't blame her. I kicked and screamed, and when it was all said and done, Benjamin loved playing with other kids. Many parents insist that daycare can provide a mentally stimulating environment beyond what can be offered at home, even with the best of intentions. Regardless, from the second he was enrolled, it seems as though he became sick with a cold or a stomach bug, all too often.

Not two weeks passed without him vomiting or coughing, in which case one of us was required to take the day off work. Fevers can be pretty scary to say the least. In fact, I suspect that the financial success of Tempra® (Baby Tylenol®), is because of this inherent, well-founded fear. Don't get me wrong, having access to fever medication is great, specifically if indeed a child's fever gets too high for comfort, without being a medical emergency. However, there's more than enough evidence suggesting that fevers are indeed a healthy bodily response to an infection that needs to be supported rather than suppressed.[1] Basically, it all comes down to enzymes.

Certain aspects of the innate immune response simply works better with a fever.[2] Have you ever wondered why you're not hungry typically while feeling feverish? It turns out, digestive enzymes function more optimally at lower temperatures compared with those implemented in supporting the immune system, during an infection. The body is ingenious in this way. It's as if the body is bringing out the 'big guns', 'tanks' even. The catch, is that these weapons of mass infectious destruction, work best at higher temperatures and require massive amounts of energy. Thus, digesting food becomes less important as the immediate task at hand, so hunger decreases and temperature rises. Remember in Star Trek, when Captain Kirk said, "Scotty, I need more power!"? Then, at the last second, Scotty diverted auxiliary power from the deflector dish to the forward shields, saving the Enterprise and quite possibly the entire galaxy, from utter annihilation. It's a matter of resource allocation. Although science has been pursuing the exact mechanisms of action, involving additional components of the innate immune response such as interleukin-1, reactive oxygen intermediates and nitric oxide production, the seemly simple concept of developing a fever, quickly becomes daunting.

Fevers are indeed scary. Thus, I don't judge anyone who jumps on medication for the purpose of reducing one. Nevertheless, seeking professional advice to help manage a fever successfully, will take advantage of all its positive attributes can offer. Generally, this includes watchful waiting along with damp cool cloths under armpits, around the neck, and over a child's back, taking thermometer readings often, thus maintaining a stable, safe temperature. I realize that it's not as easy as it sounds, as children can become extremely temperamental.

Infections typically get worse as the day progresses. Sound familiar? As a parent, it's perfect timing, isn't it? After a long, exhausting work day, parents scramble to create a last minute dinner, use whatever energy they have left for play time, followed by bath time, pj's, and bedtime, they yearn for that one hour of 'me time.' It is during 'me time,' when fevers conveniently break. You might realize the same pattern in yourself too. Think about the last time you had a cold or the flu. Was it worse in the morning or at night? Night, and here's probably why. Our stress response is protective against certain sickness symptoms.[3] Recall that cortisol is anti-inflammatory and is supposed to be at the highest in the morning. As the day progresses cortisol should decline, and with it, it's protective effects against too much inflammation. As a result, symptoms worsen. At least that's the simple way of explaining it.

The Most Important Meal of the Day

Imagine reviewing your four-point salivary cortisol test, noticing highs when there should be lows and vice versa. People often suspect that they're cortisol is too high when they have experienced tremendous amounts of stress. There's a constant feeling of being fatigued, you can't seem to lose weight; a story many of us have heard all too often. In my experience, these people may be correct in that they're cortisol is indeed elevated, but in the evening. I suspect this may be a contributing factor towards developing sleep disturbances as it's counterproductive to be responding to stress at the time of the day when you should be at your most relaxed state. I find it interesting that within the natural health industry, naturopathic doctors included, we find ourselves running towards anti-inflammatory herbs and medicines which are predicated on creating predictable, physiological responses within our adrenal glands. If cortisol is suspected as being too low, herbs and supplements are sought to stimulate the adrenals glands in an effort to increase production. The opposite is true if cortisol is too high. Yet, this goes against simply nourishing the adrenal glands, helping them respond appropriately to whatever stressors emerge. Therefore, one of the most overlooked approaches for stress management in my opinion, involves nutrient dense, whole foods. Here's why.

If the adrenal glands are over taxed for too long, as in the case of chronic stress, essentially they lose their ability to respond to stress in the same way. An analogy can be made with a car running nearly on empty. For some reason, the engine just doesn't respond quite as well, as compared to when the gas tank is full. Perhaps it's the way the fuel pump interacts with gas. I'm not sure. Either way, during chronic stress, our nutrient requirements increase, particularly with respect to certain vitamins and minerals from real, whole food. Vitamin C, certain B vitamins, protein, zinc, to name a few. During the time of the day when our adrenal glands should be responding at their peak, pumping out the most cortisol, is often where our society consumes the least amount of nutrition.

They say that breakfast is the most important meal of the day. Yet, as a society, we're bombarded with too many tasks and time limits first thing in the morning and everything seems to be rushed, all the time, doesn't it? Therefore, when it comes to satisfying that energy gap first thing, we often resort to highly refined, simple carbohydrates and sugar containing deserts, along with a warm beverages containing loads of high energy cream and sugar. Don't get me wrong, they taste fantastic and will keep you coming back for more every time. However, they are also incredible low on the nutrient density scale. Essentially, we are providing ourselves with large amounts of calories without very many nutrients. We can certainly have these treats once in a while, but certainly not every day as is the norm for a surprising amount of people. The adrenal glands require nutrition first thing in the morning to respond properly to stress, thus producing cortisol from cholesterol. Therefore, those people who have been experiencing chronic stress, yet eat this way in the morning or skip breakfast all together on a regular basis, are missing out on a key opportunity. Although we will discuss nutrient dense foods in more detail later on in this book, I propose that you begin thinking about nutrient dense foods that you can eat first thing in the morning, providing nutrition when you may need it the most. That is, low calorie foods, full of healthy nutrients. Sorry, supplements do not count.

Stress management is connected with chronic disease development through inflammation and energy metabolism, as seen through cortisol. Moreover, inflammation is an integral part of the immune system, and is both necessary and unavoidable. Adrenal fatigue is a commonly used term nowadays though not everyone validates it as a real diagnosis. In reality when the adrenals glands fail to produce adequate amounts of certain hormones, it's referred to as Adrenal Insufficiency or Addison's Disease. [4] Still, whichever way medical professionals label someone when they're stress response (or HPA axis as it's called) is working sub-optimally, to the person experiencing symptoms, it can feel all too real. The good news, is that there are incredible tools and tips available to us, that we can implement nutritionally, helping to restore adrenal health and inflammation, improving chronic disease risk factors and most importantly the way we feel. In my opinion, this most certainly involves nurturing cholesterol.

Lowering Cholesterol is Easy

Lowering cholesterol is easy. We have pharmaceutical drugs for that. What drugs concomitantly offer however, are potential unhealthy side effects. One well known example lies within the realm of statin drugs such as Lipitor® (atorvastatin), Crestor® (rosuvastatin). These HMG CoA Reductase Inhibitors, deplete an important coenzyme that helps our cells use oxygen properly in the conversion of sugar to usable energy called ATP. Coenzyme Q10, as it's called, is a widely used supplement, substantiated with literature in the coadministering with statin drugs. Further, Peter H. Langsjoen, MD, in his report found on the FDA's website, suggests the following be placed on every black box warning label on statins sold in the USA:

"Warning: HMG CoA reductase inhibitors block the endogenous biosynthesis of an essential co-factor, coenzyme Q10, required for energy production. A deficiency of coenzyme Q10 is associated with impairment of myocardial function, with liver dysfunction and with myopathies (including cardiomyopathy and congestive heart failure). All patients taking HMG CoA reductase inhibitors should therefore be advised to take 100 to 200 mg per day of supplemental coenzyme Q10."[5]

There has been a tremendous amount of research on Coenzyme Q10 in terms of its ability to improve cardiovascular health, protect cell lipid peroxidation (damage to the cell membrane)[6], and possibly protect our mitochondria from damage, which are often explained as energy producing 'factories' within our cells.[7] By depleting this coenzyme, statins can negatively affect muscle tissue in the form of myopathies, notably within the heart.. Depending on who you speak with, this is either considered common or extremely rare. Regardless, whether you take coenzyme Q10 or not, the side effects of medication is not my only concern.

Less Cholesterol Equals Less Risk; Sort Of

The most important thing to consider regarding cholesterol lowering interventions is whether reducing amounts indeed lowers risk factors for developing cardiovascular disease. On one hand, we know that less blood circulating fat and cholesterol, equates to less hypothetical chance for hardening of the arteries and/or plaque formation within their lumens. The catch twenty-two is that we need both for survival. Furthermore, if we're still consuming foods and living lifestyles that cause an imbalance in our body's ability to create and respond to inflammation, immune responses, tackle oxidative stress, and metabolize energy, then not only are we still at risk for cardiovascular disease but other forms of chronic disease, such as diabetes, hypertension, cancer, bone loss, and aging in general. For those reasons, in my opinion, lowering or even inhibiting the production of cholesterol, is not the answer. Not by a long shot.

There is no question in my mind that drugs have their place. Having access to these medications can be temporarily life saving for someone who is at a severely high risk for inflammation and cardiovascular disease risk in general (smoking, obesity, family history, previous history, etc.).

However, this is by no means an effective long term strategy. Nothing comes close to lifestyle interventions. The reason, is because they are more complex.

Comprehensive strategies using nutrition and exercise should focus specific attention on key factors directly responsible for damaging cholesterol in the first place, resulting in a danger to our quality of life. We must not fall into a common trap of solely keeping an eye on cholesterol blood levels, but rather our mission needs to address the root cause of the problem, helping cholesterol to work properly. Have you heard of Dyson vacuum cleaners? Dyson's an engineer, realizing that most vacuum cleaners have never really worked well in the first place, as one of their big problems has always been a gradual loss of suction. So, Dyson spent time and energy redesigning the vacuum cleaner from the ground up, investing a machine that never loses suction. His motto, is "I just think things should work properly". I, much as Dyson with his vacuum cleaner, think that cholesterol, our inflammatory and stress response, the way we metabolize energy, should work properly.

In acquiring a basic level of understanding now of what cholesterol does and why we absolutely need it, we can finally begin shifting our focus in examining what really causes damage to cholesterol from a dietary/lifestyle point of view. I'm going to show you exactly how I would evaluate my own diet; more specifically, what I would look for in terms of maintaining healthy cholesterol levels, but far more important, good health of cholesterol itself.

Chapter 5:

The King of All Vegetables

I owe everything I know in terms of naturopathic medicine to my Mom, Evelin Horovitz. If not for the simple fact that after over a decade studying, practicing, and immersing myself both within the naturopathic profession as well as the natural health industry of which I have fallen in love with, I realize now more than ever that she was absolutely right about everything, all along. "Broccoli is the king of all vegetables?" she has always maintained. My Mom is a magnificent woman. After losing her father Wilhelm Friedlieb, who I'm named after, to colon cancer when she was merely 11, she helped my grandmother raise my uncle and has always carried with her and onto myself and three brothers, the value of life, as she knows all too well how quickly it can be taken from each of us.

It's a horrible fear; death of a loved one or even oneself. One which I admit to be living with even now. Perhaps that's a real truth as to why I have wanted to pursue a career in medicine from such an early age. They were best friends, Mom and my grandfather. They even had their own secret language, and as the theory goes, my grandmother was jealous. For him to be ripped away from his family when he was in his mere 50's was incredibly tragic and has devastated the family since, as I'm sure you can relate. The reason I'm sharing this with you, is because I too have an idea what severe loss as well as dying far too young, looks like. Being in your 50's or 60's can be scary, in relation to cardiovascular disease. I suppose one reason, is that heart attack risk as well as severity tend to be most aggressive after the age of 65, with women being even more likely than men to die within a few weeks.[1]

Perhaps the greatest tragedy of all, depending how you look at it, is that cardiovascular disease in many respects is preventable. The American Heart Association tells me that "A healthy diet is one of the best weapons you have to fight CVD)." Who am I to argue with the American Heart Association? "Look," my Mom says. "There are many things that we just don't know. Some things you just can't prevent and are out of your control. In fact, most things in this world, we can't control. The two things that I know for sure, and the two rare things that I know we CAN control, are:

What Mom Knows for Sure:

- We only have one body
- We die alone as no one else is going to step into the grave with us.

What Mom Knows We Can Control:

- How much we exercise
- What we put into our body (what we eat)

For over 40 years, my Mom has been working out. If you're saying "good for your Mom", you're absolutely right. In fact, great for my Mom. She's been waking up at around 6am, heading off to "the club", looking forward to 'her time,' consisting of about 30 minutes of cardio on the treadmill and then an hour spinning class, followed by either stretching or core strengthening exercises. Although she along with a growing movement of healthusiasts look forward to exercise, it's common knowledge that not everyone sees eye to eye, to say the least. "It's boring", "it's hard", "that's too early", "she's crazy", and "why does she put herself through all that?" These are the comments she has ignored for decades, way before exercise was fashionable the way it is today. In terms of food, she has focused on maintaining a mostly vegetarian plate with a little bit of lean meat or fish, and a small amount of complex carbs. She rarely drinks alcohol and growing up, there was never an occasion where we had alcohol served at our house under any circumstance. There's more.

Salad is absolutely her favorite food and most of the time when she goes out to eat, she orders an overpriced one to boot. When I say overpriced, I suppose that in my opinion, $18 plus tax and tip for someone to just rip open one of the pre-made salad bags and throw it on a plate with some pre-packaged dressing or EVO, balsamic, and S & P, is more than ridiculous and I'd go as far as to say even insulting in some way. Especially when I can order something of real value such as a mouth-watering, sizzling steak almost! "You don't get it!" she exclaims, convincing me to order the same thing. "You're paying so that you don't over eat. Also, to avoid that 'blah' feeling most people get after eating a really heavy meal." When Mom's right, she's right.

My Mom has high cholesterol. You heard right. Can you believe it? HIGH. She's was diagnosed years ago as having familial hypercholesterolemia. Her liver produces more cholesterol than the average person. It's actually more common than you might think and for all I know, you may have it yourself. A few years ago, while studying naturopathic medicine no less, I was seduced into cracking open a bag of potato chips. Now let's for a moment pretend that these chips weren't laced with MSG and genetically modified corn isolates. Hi, my name is Robert and I'm addicted to potato chips. Once I start, I can't stop. Seriously, it's disgusting. If you place one of those massive Costco chip bags in front of me without pouring some in a small bowl or literally tell me when to stop, I will crush it whole heartedly (no pun intended). Talk about that 'blah' feeling. That's precisely why they shouldn't be in the house in the first place.

What started as a potato chip binge after exams, continued into exploring the wonderful world of Burger King® and oh boy do I love a good Whopper®. Do you remember the days when if you walked into a BK literally asking for a "Whopper®" instead of a one or two patty burger, you received a discount or a paper crown? After engulfing a double Whopper® a few days prior to my annual checkup with my family physician, guess what? High cholesterol and blood pressure. By the way, Burger King® shouldn't receive blame here, but rather high consumption of processed, fatty, meats, cheeses, and refined carbohydrates within 'fast food', generally speaking. Although they both normalized over the next few months, my readings were scary nevertheless. The experience offered me personal insight behind the saying 'you're only as good as you feel.' In reality, that's not often the case. Heart disease, after all, is the silent killer.

If you're overweight and can't breathe or move the same as you once could, there is a dramatic impact on your quality of life. When being out of shape affects your ability to function on a daily basis, certainly the impact is dramatic and noticeable. In this way, much as in a failed relationship, where the signs are often present for a long period of time, gone unnoticed by one or both parties, heart disease and chronic disease progression too have their warnings. Nevertheless, and far too often, just as relationships end, so do people inevitably ignore, put off, or simply aren't aware of these warnings until it's far too late. The good news regarding cholesterol is that concrete lab results are easy to access. Inquiring with your doctor about a lipid profile, will surely impress.

If you're like me, having a blood test isn't exactly on your favourite things to do, list. Instead you'll wait until your doctor insists. The syringe feels like dark age technology, doesn't it? I'll never forget my phlebotomy training. The thought of using needles, possibly causing someone pain, sent a shiver down my spine each and every time, regardless of how necessary it may have seemed. When a 7-year-old girl with a fear of needles and "difficult veins" showed up with her protective parents, all eyes were on me for the blood draw, and let me tell you that as a student, sweat pouring down my face was an understatement. After pausing to collect my thoughts, I heard for the millionth time, my supervisor's only recycled joke "I'd be more scared if you weren't afraid of needles" (only to start laughing at her own act). Needless to say, the draw was performed perfectly this specific time and the feeling of relief was overwhelming as I saw her smile. "It wasn't so bad", she admitted.

At the time of writing this, a woman by the name of Elizabeth Holmes may change blood draws forever, with her tiny drop approach.[2] Imagine being capable of performing multiple blood tests using merely a fraction of the previous standard blood volume. By going back to the drawing board and literally redesigning each test to accommodate a smaller amount of blood, not only has she become America's youngest billionaire, but more importantly, her company Theranos may have changed the face of blood tests as we know it.[3] Until this technology becomes mainstream, unfortunately many tests we use still depend on blood but let me at least reassure you that the lipid profile is pretty routine and no sweat off your doctor's back. Here is what it includes:

Typical Cholesterol Lipid Panel:

- LDL Cholesterol
- HDL Cholesterol
- Total Cholesterol
- Total: HDL Ratio
- Triglycerides

You should find reference ranges often located next to test result numbers, thus placing into context where your results lie. An example of a test result is: 210 (100-300 units). In this case, it means the following: 210 is in between the reference range of 100-300 so is interpreted as being within normal range. Conversely, if the test result read 50, this would be indicative of a low value, with 400 being obscenely elevated, does that make sense? As a more challenging read, I have been preview to many lab reports where someone's values read incredibly close to the outer edge of the reference range. For example; 102 (100-300 units) where a note was written as "normal". In my opinion, this is too close for comfort and although technically within range, this merits a low value interpretation, with the whole person placed into context. If you have any of your tests on you right now, you may want to have a second look as if your values lie extremely close to the outer areas of a reference range, you may wish to inquire further with your doctor.

Lipid panels are more complex and in all honesty laboratory diagnosis in general can be incredibly difficult, often requiring years of experience before even the most highly trained professionals become experts. Lipid panels, oddly enough do not have single reference ranges. Instead, doctors must spend time evaluating a patients overall cardiovascular disease risk as being low, moderate, or high, taking into consideration variables such as age, gender, total and HDL cholesterol, blood pressure level, medications, smoking status, family history, and even their patient's own history such as whether they've had previous heart attacks or strokes. Depending which level doctors suspect a patient fits best with, their lipid panel values will then be placed into appropriate context.

The following values are from The College of Family Physicians of Canada's website for your viewing pleasure.[4]

- An LDL cholesterol level of less than 3.0 mmol/L is best

- An HDL above 1.0 mmol/L is best

- If your risk is low, your LDL cholesterol should be less than 5.0 mmol/L and total cholesterol to HDL-C ratio should be less than 6.0

- If your risk is moderate, your LDL cholesterol should be less than 3.5 mmol/L and total cholesterol to HDL-C ratio should be less than 5

- If your risk is high, your LDL cholesterol should be less than 2.0 mmol/L and total cholesterol to HDL-C ratio should be less than 4.0

- An HDL cholesterol level of less than 1.0 mmol/L means you're at higher risk for heart disease.

- If you have diabetes, your LDL should be less than 2.0 mmol/L.

- If you've already had a heart attack your LDL needs to be less than 2.0 mmol/L.

Chapter 6:

Moderation Through the Eyes of the Beholder

In addition to blood work, Naturopathic Doctors will often prescribe a diet diary at the end of a patient's first visit. However, completing beforehand is an excellent way to help save time and money. I'll go as far as to say that this is probably one of the most valuable tips I can possibly offer you. In comparison to most visits with a Medical Doctor, spending an hour with your ND may seem like an abundance of time, yet flies by quicker than you might expect. Since building a strong foundation is paramount in developing an individualized, comprehensive, holistic treatment plan, most of a first visit is taken up by the ND obtaining a full case history. Unlike a 6 or 7 minute visit that most people are accustomed to with their Medical Doctor, a more in depth naturopathic visits not only allow for, but encourage patients to ask questions and truly engage in their wellbeing. Needless to say, one piece of homework almost guaranteed to be prescribed by the end, is indeed a diet diary to be completed for the follow up visit, usually scheduled one to two weeks following. It is at this time, where ND's will analyze and review this incredibly valuable tool with their patient to empower positive change as far as nutrition is concerned.

Dr. Rob's Diet Diary Example:

Time	Sunday	Monday	Tuesday	Wednesday	Thursday	Friday	Saturday
9:00 am	3 eggs, oven roasted potatoes (1 tsp olive oil), 2 sausages, 2 peameal bacon, 9 oz coffee, 2 tbsp cream, 1 tsp organic cane sugar, 1 slice light rye, 1/2 tsp butter, 1 tsp olive oil.						
11:00 am	500 ml smoothie (collared greens, 1/2 banana, 2 tbsp hemp hearts)						
1:00 pm	300 ml chicken soup, tuna sandwich (light rye), 1 tbsp mayo, cucumber and tomato, 250 ml water						
3:00 pm	30 min cardio, 45 min weights, 600 ml water						
5:30 pm							
7:30 pm							
9:00 pm							

I can't speak highly enough of diet diaries. Filling out what you've eaten during the course of a week is a great way to visually see where you may have succeeded as well as fallen short of your goals. I suggest labelling specific meals as well as times. Adding information regarding water/beverage as well as specific exercises and duration, offer substantial value in my opinion. For example, sets and reps if you're lifting weights, and minutes if you're jogging, biking, or even going outside to walk your dogs. It's not a perfect system by any means. Often you might catch yourself having a 'bad week' and that's more than fine. Still, write everything down. You just went on a cruise? You had relatives from a distant country visit? You celebrated a birthday or a religious holiday? You had a huge amount of frozen food in the house that you just couldn't let go to waste? I completely understand. These things happen to the best of us as life is dynamic that way.

Still, I encourage you to write it all down. You went to McDonalds® on the way to The Beer Store® as it was right next door and the 'golden arches' were staring at you? No problem, write it down. Your spouse tied you to a chair and made you eat a Dairy Queen® Blizzard® because that's your way of finally spending time together? Write it down. Your child received an A+ on an exam and you rewarded with a trip to the all you can eat buffet? "No problemo!" Jot everything down on paper. It's only one week. How bad can it be, right?

I found that while creating my own diet diary, and I've done this several times for different reasons, it was truly an eye opener each and every time. What I find most surprising is how convincing we can get when we're trying to sell ourselves on how well we did during prior weeks. After all; on a day to day basis, we are dealing with all of the complexities of life and its relative stressors, aren't we? Work, kids, health, traffic, you name it. There are so many ways that eating both fast and unhealthy can feel fantastic in the moment, am I right or am I right?! It's late afternoon and you hadn't eaten since breakfast. Here, wait, let me set this scene up properly.

It's winter, someone had the flu, and you didn't sleep. Your morning started off with you running behind, and breakfast consisted of a bar in the car as you were waiting for your windshield to dethaw. Now it's 3:00pm or so and you have 20 minutes until your next appointment. You're absolutely famished. In that moment you just think 'ugh, why didn't I bring my own food? Again, I'm going to have to eat out.' Let's analyze; you're already aware of that fact that eating out isn't healthy. Of course it's not. It's harder to control what's in your food; sodium content, fats, sugar, freshness. You end up grabbing a sub because it's at least the 'healthier' option relative to burgers, fries, and a sugary soft drink. Ok fine, you ordered a diet iced tea because at least there's tea in it and they used aspartame instead of sugar, saving on calories.

Living in these moments, means using effort and will power, and for many of us, requires mental struggle to an extent. Choosing the sub over what you really want, which is a greasy burger with fries. Yes, it's a struggle as you're going against the grain regardless of whether eating a sub is indeed the healthiest decision possible. I completely understand. Overcoming these 'struggles', require will power and feels great regardless of whether these choices includes the better of the worse, at times. I suppose in these situations it truly requires honesty. We need to be honest with ourselves if we are to succeed in achieving our goals. Little things add up over time and if you falter, that's fine, no judgment here, but when you don't reach your goals, and you aren't surprised, how does that feel? I've been there many times and let me just volunteer here; it doesn't feel good. Not in the slightest. A diet diary can dramatically help you stay focused, but more importantly, help you remain honest with yourself.

Eating healthy is easy in concept; common, nutrient dense, whole foods. However, most of us fall in the trap of 'moderation', which should really be the theme of this book, I think. Moderation obviously means 'once in a blue moon,' but it's just so subjective, isn't it? "Meh, I've been good these last few days. I can probably afford to eat cheese pizza. It's just one slice. I'll make it up tomorrow. Everything in moderation." In reality of course, the days leading up to this pizza craving probably consisted of a fair bit of food which were unproductive as far as health goals are concerned. A few handfuls of Chicago Mix popcorn (caramel popcorn and cheese flavoured popcorn married in one delicious bag) late at night. A slice of bread, butter, and cheese for breakfast one early morning. No matter which way I slice it, my diet diary keeps me honest, if nothing else. When you look at your diet diary, and if you know what it is you're looking for, then 'moderation' has a whole new meaning, not to anyone else but you. Logging, reviewing, and improving my weekly diet chart, log, diary, calendar, or whatever you want to call it, has helped empower and place me in the driver seat. As we dive into specifics of what to look for using this incredible tool, I hope that I can help you achieve the same.

Chapter 7:

Carbs Gone Wild

Carbs are hot and I'm not just referring to your spaghetti dinner. Breads, cereals, crackers, and some of the tastiest snacks out there have been surrounded by a media frenzy, haven't they? In fact, carbs everywhere have been running scared like turkeys before Thanksgiving, ever since the Gluten Free craze has gained international acclaim. As the topic of weight loss has long made the headlines, carbs, being an energy source that can lead to weight gain, had to go. Really? Well, no; not really.

To throw you a curve ball, bodybuilders will tell you that carbs are unbelievably important in building muscle mass, which is the 'anti-fat,' as muscles are energy (sugar, carbs, fat) burning machines. Wait a minute. Stop the clock. Carbs for muscle? Yes! In fact, some argue that carbs may be more important in building muscle than even protein to a degree. Not only are carbs widely available and inexpensive, but I mean; who can resist the smell of freshly baked bread? My Dad surely can't and I'll be honest here; the apple doesn't fall far from the tree on this one.

My wife's grandmother makes something called "pischki" (pish-key) and although Dad has never tried it, I have no doubt that it would make his top 5, easily. Basically, it's a homemade donut, and yes, its fried in oil and they eat it first thing in the morning, dipped in sugar, and paired up with a hot cuppa Joe with 10% cream. As far as the taste buds go, let's just say that I spent most of that last sentence daydreaming and drooling. When reviewing someone's week's worth diet diary, one of the first things that I look at is what type of carbs they are eating and how often. There are several reasons for this.

The major point of maintaining healthy cholesterol levels is prevention of heart disease, leading to heart attacks and strokes. For some reason, although the literature is absolutely confusing, conflicting, and controversial, it seems to me that energy management is truly the link between all theories. Energy from our diet in the form of sugar, carbs, fat, and yes, even protein, is digested and enters the blood stream to be transported to our cells, where it's required for basically everything we do. Whatever is not used, gets stored ingeniously in the form of fat. I seldom think of just how much energy it takes to perform simple activities of daily living such as smiling and laughing, to digesting our food, to firing neurons in our brains, and even our hearts relentlessly contracting and pump blood effortlessly for a lifetime.

The process of going back and forth between storing and then requiring and using energy, seems to create 'rust' in the body in the form of oxidative damage.[1] It also appears that the longer and the more often fat travels through the blood, the greater chance that it will become oxidized either by inflammation within the artery or by some other factor, which in turn contributes to plaque formation over long periods of time.[2,3] Consequently, the narrowing of a blood vessel's inner lumen compromises circulation while also increasing the chance of plaque dislodging, flowing down stream and possibly blocking blood flow, causing either a myocardial infarction in the heart or a stroke in the brain.

Forget about all the bad press you've heard about carbs. Forget about the grains that lurk in our brains, or the refined wheat that lazes around in our belly, only to make us sleepy and grant us that beautiful 'food coma' after a delicious second helping of pasta the way "mama used to make". Carbs are an energy source, but only if they're used wisely. If you're piling on more carbs because they taste great or you're bored, they inevitably store as fat, just in case one day you decide to get off that office chair of yours and explore the idea of maybe going for a "walk" (window shopping) with a colleague. In that case, I hate to be the bearer of bad news, but excess carbs just aren't for you. What do I mean by excess? That my friend is a great question!

Everything in moderation, right? I don't disagree. Here's the thing; if you're gaining weight or if you are generally overweight and have a difficult time slimming down or maintaining your optimal weight, you may be storing more energy than you're using by a long shot, and you aren't eating carbs in moderation relative to what your body is using them for. Does that make sense? What if you just simply have a slower metabolism and just don't burn fat as easily as someone else? Perhaps you have an under functioning thyroid gland. For those reason and more, I hear you and it's not easy. However, if your body isn't using energy as efficiently, there's very little reason to consume more energy than what your body is using, wouldn't you agree? Is it possible to eat more, exercise more, and still lose body fat? Absolutely; bodybuilders eat ten plus meals per day at times, gain weight in terms of muscle mass, however appear leaner, regardless. That said, for most of us who aren't bodybuilders, moderation is moderation, customized to how your mind and body will respond. The way I see it; it's reasonable for us to take in about as much as we're using. Therefore, gaining weight in the form of extra body fat, as a result, is a common sense way of telling us that we're eating too much energy relative to our fitness level. Let me put it to you a different way.

When evaluating someone's diet diary for healthy cholesterol management, my job is first to ascertain where the majority of their calories are coming from, because it makes the most sense to look at total risk factors for cardiovascular disease, and not exclusively dietary intake of cholesterol itself. Obesity is a major risk factor and so calories have to come into play. In my experience, the majority of calories come from carbs then sugar, and finally fat. It's not surprising really, as for the last few decades we have been conditioned to replace saturated fats such as creams and butters, with other "low fat" or "no fat" ingredients/additives, which often are in the form of highly processed, refined, carbs and sugars.

Researchers all over the globe compare diets such as the Mediterranean, with respective intake ratios of saturated to unsaturated fats (monounsaturated and polyunsaturated) to carbohydrate. Although the literature is often confusing, I am impressed, discovering that certain studies have really taken into consideration not only regenerative benefits versus detriments, but have placed into context, human behaviour. When we traded in our deep fried peanut butter and banana sandwiches, and bacon wrapped chicken wings for foods without saturated fats, what foods did we choose, and was cardiovascular disease risk reduced? The answer, was pretty much that we replaced them with increased carbs and sugar, with an overwhelming result of, "not really". Replacing saturated fats with 'good fats' (poly and mono-unsaturated) received a gold star for decreasing LDL cholesterol, but on the flip side, HDL also plummeted.[4] Replacing saturated fat with increased refined carbohydrates, increased risk of artery hardening, fat metabolism imbalance, decrease in insulin's ability to work optimally (increased insulin resistance), and obesity, which included increased triglycerides, LDL cholesterol, total cholesterol, and decreased HDL cholesterol.[5] Not good! Replacing carbs with healthy fats however showed improvement in all these areas.

In terms of moderation, does your breakfast consist mostly of toast with jam, cereal, or maybe just a cup of coffee? Do you add sugar to your coffee? One lump or two? What's for lunch? Slice of pizza, a sub, or a sandwich with a few pieced of thinly sliced, highly processed, preserved, salted, nitrate infested cold cuts between two fairly thick pieces of bread, having many of the same credentials? Do you shop at Costco® so that you can buy those massive boxes of low fat bars for the road or as a mid-day 'healthy snack'? By the way, I love Costco®, and granola bars truly aren't that unhealthy when compared with other vices such my potato chip addiction. However, I'm inquiring about the sheer amount of sugar and carbs consumed from the moment you wake up until your last meal before bed. Furthermore, I'm trying to build context in terms of how much energy your body really needs from food, based on the amount of physical activity performed on a particular day. When you finally get home from a long day of work, what portion of your plate is taken up by carbs? My guess is large.

Tip: I typically recommend (and I didn't make this up; it was taught in school) that a great rule of thumb, is to consider 1 plate of food = 1/4 protein, 1/4 carb, 1/2 veggies. Plus, if you're reaching for seconds, keep to that same ratio. What is often found is that people tend to reach for just carbs the next time around. I never understood that personally as I always think of the meat as the being the more expensive and succulent portion of the meal. Different strokes, I suppose.

It's funny; I really want to share the difference between complex and simple carbs, but I don't want to be one of those guys who leads you to believe that simple carbs are bad while complex are good, because it's not that easy. I really believe that in the grand scheme of things, total carb intake still needs to be taken into consideration. In other words, just because you think that it's better to order whole wheat buns for your sub or even kamut and spelt for you savvy shoppers out there, doesn't mean you can eat a ton of it, carte blanche. Whether you are eating the regular, white flour kind or more wholesome options, excess carbohydrates (based on your bodies usage; exercise, etc.), no matter how nutritious, will still become stored as fat in the form of triglycerides, which inevitably travel through the blood stream to potentially become oxidized, contributing to heart disease risk. Still, there is a profound difference.

The carbs and sugar that you acquire in your white bread 'pb and j' sandwich, become digested much quicker than whole grain counterparts, spiking your blood sugar as well as insulin production, which over long periods of time increases risk for diabetes and thus heart disease. Conversely, higher fibre, whole grain breads, takes much longer to digest. Instead of blood sugar spiking all at once, whole, unprocessed grains digest slower, with smaller, more regulated blood sugar spurts, resulting in longer, more sustained energy. Key observations when shopping for breads include processed ingredients, which I'll elaborate upon later in the grocery walk through section of this book. Otherwise, generally speaking, 1-2g of fiber per average slice is considered poor, while 3-5g is excellent.

Chapter 8:

Fat & Happy

If lowering or maintaining healthy cholesterol levels are a goal of yours, having an idea of how much of your fat intake is cholesterol rich, is a great starting point. Fat in general is also a pretty heavy source of calories and so if weight loss is part of your plan, being aware of where the bulk of it is coming from, has merit. Since cholesterol is found in animal fat, dairy, meat, and eggs are the first places where I look. High fat containing dairy products, include cream in a person's coffee (5%, 10%, 18%), sour cream, butter, lard, and cheese (cream cheese is still cheese [sorry]). Right away, I highlight these items on a person's diary to emphasize how often they're consuming them. Pop quiz: how much cheese is a person with high cholesterol allowed per day while on a dietary restriction plan? Although I'm not giving out medical advice, here, I was taught to stay conservatively within a 1 cm by 1 cm cube, which is literally about the size of one of those little samples of cheeses that you see on toothpicks in grocery stores. Yah, I know. So in my book, its best not to have any, as once you have a little bit, if you're like me, you may not be able to hold back.

I absolutely love coffee. I love the smell and the culture. The thought of bean to cup, intrigues me. What goes into growing the beans followed by the incredible array of steps taken prior to reaching a roaster, only to finally arrive at store shelves months later, is fascinating. Finally, by the time it gets into the hands of consumers, of course the final product is marketed as 'fresh,' when in reality, it couldn't be farther from the truth, could it? It's been a hobby of mine for quite some time now to purchase coffee from local roasters who have direct relationships with farmers. That's one side of it. The other involves brewing methods themselves. Like a bunch of geeks in science class, coffee culture investigates proper temperature, pressure, timing, and precise amounts of coffee, weighed using scales. Super expensive grinding machines are evaluated for their consistency and precision down to the micron. This is all with the intention of accomplishing uniform bean particle size, while maintaining the right amount of heat, all in name of enjoying that perfect cup. Of course it's not really about the cup, is it? Probably the more inspiring aspect of coffee culture, is its connection between nature, people, and passion. I just love it.

"Cream in coffee is like putting ketchup on an expensive steak". This is a quote that I read recently (source unknown). I spent $6.00 for a cup of siphoned coffee a few months ago. It so reminds me of a high school science experiment involving Bunsen burners. Remember those? Wow, are they theatrical. In true essence, I'm convinced that siphoned coffee is no different than immersion brewed coffee, but to be sure, I'll have to inquire further at my next visit to Trebilcock Coffee Roasters in Pickering, Ontario. Like a rookie, I asked the barista how he takes his coffee. You should see the look on his face. It was as if I committed coffee blasphemy. He said "Please, please, I beg you. Please don't pollute my coffee by adding anything to it. It was meant to be enjoyed the way it is". I took his advice and of course it was really good. The level of acidity was low, the bitterness truly gone. It was a really smooth, great cuppa Joe. Between you and I, it was just good, but you know what would have made it great? Yes, that's right; cream! 10% all the way and just enough to change the colour to a nice brown, wouldn't you agree?

It's amazing how you can truly get used to something over time. At home, because of my Mom's high cholesterol we drank skim milk. Once I lived on my own, I upgraded to 2% and it made a world of a difference. Then, when I met my wife and saw that her family used 5% and 10% cream, my taste buds were dancing. If you're using cream in your tea or coffee and you're concerned about your cholesterol or weight, cutting back to 2% is something that I have recommended to many. It just makes sense, doesn't it? I empathize with your taste buds completely, for what its worth. Believe me, I won't lie to you and tell you that it tastes the same, but you will truly get used to it. Your coffee will still taste fantastic, and besides, if you are a true coffee drinker (which I suppose I'm not), you'll drink it without anything added whatsoever.

Growing up in a household where we didn't usually have very fatty meats, whenever my brothers and I would 'treat' ourselves to deep fried chicken, or a Tuesday night, cheap chicken wing deal, we knew innately that these foods were horrible for cholesterol. I was amazed at how many of my high cholesterol patients ate these foods and more, yet were (or acted) surprised when I pointed them out as red flags. I suppose my brothers and I grew up with the idea of maintaining healthy cholesterol through diet and exercise, but for many, the concept is foreign. Either that, or they were caught with their 'hand in the cookie jar' and a natural reaction to look surprised. I choose to give them the benefit of the doubt.

Not Your Average Chicken

Deep fried food is so bad for us yet tastes so unbelievably good. Is it because of the high fat content? I mean, that's part of it for sure. There's actually quite a bit of debate regarding the issue of fat. It really isn't as easy as just making a blanket statement such as "fat is bad for you", because in reality it's not. Fat is actually incredibly good for us even in the case of saturated animal fat as I'll come back to this a little later. Perhaps just as important or maybe even more important than the type and amounts of fat one consumes, is respective cooking methods.

Have you tasted fried chicken down in New Orleans? This my friend, is not your fast food, run of the mill, deep fried. Despite my previous belief, I quickly learned that fried chicken truly isn't 'just deep fried chicken' until indulged in southern cooking, let me tell you! The batter isn't the lumpy, textured, crunchy kind, that we have at most places here in Ontario (not that I know from experience). While traveling down there, I found batter consistent with that of good fish and chips, but thin. You know how fish and chips batter tends to be crispy on the outside yet so thick that as soon as you crisp through that outside layer, it sort of tastes like a pancake inside? This wasn't 'battery' on the inside. No sir/ma'am. In New Orleans, it was thin and crispy all the way through and then the meat, ever so juicy. The crisp was unlike anything I've tasted before. Furthermore, the light colour typically seen in these northern neck of the woods, was nowhere to be found. Instead, a dark brown probably from staying in the fryer just a tad bit longer, prevailed. Served with collard greens and homemade mac 'n cheese; it was to die for. I thought it was pretty comical in a way that collard greens are some of the healthiest things out there, and I enjoy them in my green smoothies regularly as a matter of fact. Not these collard greens, however. No, these greens were doused in butter, laced with salt, and cooked until they just seemed to melt in your mouth.

Besides the shier amount of calories contained in such a meal, the real dangers probably lie in the actual cooking method itself! Have you ever wondered how many calories are in a tablespoon of fat? It's about 120kcal. Imagine dunking a battered, super fatty piece of meal (chicken thighs or legs with the skin on - massive amount of fat), only to completely soak in as much as it can like a Canadian taking in the rays of the sun during our only two months of summer warmth. When that gargantuan amount of fat per plate is heated at high temperatures as when being deep fried, the fat oxidizes thus changing. It becomes brown in colour, doesn't it? If you fry bacon, the same thing happens.

When white coloured chicken fat, begins turning brown, crisping up, it changes into a more dangerous version of itself as far as chronic disease is concerned. This is true for not only saturated animal fats but all fat really. In fact, unsaturated plant oils, are in many ways even more susceptible to oxidation, generating harmful chemicals. These advanced lipid oxidation end products (ALEs) as they are called, are not only toxic to cells structurally, but genetically as well, through possible mutations within our DNA.[1,2] This damage is widespread, affecting the liver, kidney, lung, gut, and so the cardiovascular system is not the only concern when it comes to fat, or rather oxidized fat.

While dangerous chemical compounds are created during the cooking process in general, deep frying and other extremely high heat methods are the worst, however not everyone cares. In fact, I must admit; when I pull apart a fresh bag of deep fried potato chips and take a whiff, somehow (and conveniently so) my brain completely forgets about the all of the toxins, which are about to be absolutely devoured. Many people take the position, that since we're bombarded by chemicals anyway, they will not be scared into living an overly cautious lifestyle.

Instead, they choose to indulge in the foods that they love, as we only live once. I'm not arguing either, as they're absolutely right.

With the shier amount of toxins ranging from air pollution from factories and cars, to toxins such as fluoride[3] in our water supply, to harmful perfluorochemicals often being emitted from our household carpets, clothes, mattresses, and some food packaging[4], to even floor lacquers, it's amazing that we can even function at all. Our bodies are pretty resilient however, and we're able to detox much of the chemical burden. Still, should we not try to minimize as much as possible? Consider all of the health conditions that we as a species are burdened with. Many are linked to inflammation and immune, as well as hormonal dysfunction, and with respect to having high cholesterol and overall risk for cardiovascular disease risk, the same applies.[5]

Highly oxidized fat interacts with the immune system inside our arteries, causing havoc; fat to the fire, so to speak. In some areas of arteries, vessel walls may be healthy and normal, in which case this oxidized, changed fat might still cause damage over time as it passes through. Other parts of an artery however, may have a mini 'war zone' periodically, caused by an infection or a situation whereby the immune system creates inflammation (the fire: fluid buildup, cellular debris, an army of white blood cells, inflammatory proteins, etc.), possibly damaging that section of the artery. What happens if oxidized fat flows through that area of inflammation within an artery? Although we don't know for sure, we think the likely answer is plaque formation, or the process thereof. There are many possible sequences of events involving foam cell generation, and I won't bore you with all of the theories. However, the common link appears to involve oxidized fat and inflammation, ultimately leading to hardening of the arteries and plaque formation, increasing risk of developing a future possible heart attack or stroke, or worse; death.

Cooking method is definitely something I always look at within a diet diary. Generally speaking, heating any oil at high temperatures is a red flag and should be avoided at all times. Please don't mistake what I'm saying as under cooking foods such as raw meats. Absolutely not. Meats should still be cooked to their specified, recommended internal temperatures that are typically listed on the label, especially if grocery store bought. That said, I'm recommending that you be patient with your food, if you aren't already.

Before placing oil on a frying pan, it's common for many to pre-heat the pan on high, speeding up the process so that when they place food to be cooked, they're rewarded with that beautiful sizzle, without sitting around waiting, am I right? It's this method of cooking that's more common around households these days than deep frying, as I have to ask; do you actually own a deep fryer? I would get rid of it, pronto. The general rule of thumb when cooking on a frying pan is to never cook on higher temperatures than medium, which is about a number 5-6 on most stovetops. It takes a little longer for the pan to heat up, that's true, but you are less likely to scorch the cooking oil as well as fats naturally contained within your food in the first place, causing significant oxidation. You'll know if you've over heated your food if you see browning, crisping, or smoking. I'm recommending that you avoid this as much as possible so long as your goal is to reduce risk of cardiovascular disease and promote lifelong wellness.

The Sizzle in Your Steak

Like many, I'm a fan of the Food Network. After all; watching chefs create incredibly brilliant dishes out of exotic food combinations, is inspiring and mouth-watering at the same time. While living in residence during my third year of naturopathic medical school, although we had a satellite connection, for some reason only 3 channels worked well. One was the food network and the other two were both day time talk shows. As a student, trying to eat healthy for the most part and cooking my own food, I learned quite a bit about cooking techniques, simply from watching and enjoyed television. I still do. In my viewing experience, many meat preparations call for searing over high heat as well as using copious amounts of seasoning (salt and pepper), offering fantastic flavour, but aren't necessarily healthy. In fact the World Health Organization strongly recommends reducing sodium intake for blood pressure and risk of cardiovascular disease and coronary heart disease in adults to 5g/day of salt.[6] 6g of table salt is about a teaspoon so pretty much about 90% of a teaspoon is what your daily intake is recommended at. Imagine all of the salt contained in many of the store bought sauces we buy, alone.

There's nothing tastier than a nicely marbled rib steak if prepared right. Chefs on television taught me the following: place a frying pan on high heat, meanwhile coating the meat in olive oil, and then add coarse sea salt and freshly ground black pepper liberally to all areas of the meat. Then, only once the pan is super-hot, place the meat to hear a dramatic sizzle. Note: if you're concerned about the drying effect seasoning can have on meat, leaving for 45 minutes prior to cooking will allow for moisture to return within the steak. Depending on how thick the cut of meat is, the longer or shorter the duration will be. Approximately 2-3 minutes later, the steak is turned over and your incredible job is evident by a crispy, seared layer, screaming of flavour. The idea is that by heating one side of the meat at high temperatures briefly and browning it (the sear), you seal off the ability for juices to escape. Not to mention, the delicious flavours that you create for you and your compadres. Once searing all sides, I was encouraged to drop the temperature down to low and cover the oven safe pan with a lid, continuing to cook at 350 degrees for about 10 minutes, achieving my preferred medium rare.

After searing, many will then add a little bit of wine to deglaze the pan. Adding a little bit of butter and freshly ground pepper will only enhance this 'sauce'. It's absolutely delicious. Needless to say, I empathize whole heartedly with anyone who it difficult to give up this method of cooking.

While 'once in a while' might be obvious to some, its personal and subjective. When reading your diet diary and eyeballing for the items you think involve deep frying or heating on high, you may be surprised as to how often you are actually consuming foods prepared in this manner. Is it 2-3 times per week? Does that sound like 'once in a while' to you? I'm suggesting to reduce it as much as possible, which truly means just that; as much as possible. Particularly if reducing cardiovascular disease risk is your goal, which it certainly is if you are concerned about high cholesterol and have the intention of promoting healthy cholesterol, lifelong.

Chapter 9:

The More I Learn About Olives

I find little reason not to be absolutely head over heels in love with olive oil. For starters, who doesn't absolutely love dunking freshly baked bread in some high quality olive oil and balsamic vinegar before the entrée? I'm always impressed at how truly serious many people take this timeless necessity. I've had the pleasure of enjoying many conversations on the subject and learned that you can often tell whether a company is providing a good quality product by the label as well as the colour and bottle type, and then of course the different nuances. Much in the same way a good wine is judged, olive oil competitions around the world take quality to a whole new level in terms of complexity, commitment, and passion.

I am no connoisseur by any means, but olive oil certainly has its fair share of health benefits. Looking for "extra virgin, first cold press" or "first press solely by mechanical means" on the label, is a good start. This means that the olives have been minimally processed, or in fact hardly processed at all, including the level of heat, which can sometimes occur in manufacturing. I've read that the best way to judge an oil is simply to taste it. Olive Oil Times, suggests placing a small amount in a little glass. Then, warm the glass with one hand and cover with the other, while bringing your nose closer to sense all of the incredible aromas. It put a smile on my face, reading their comments regarding the flavour profiles. Apparently, the aromas should "remind you of things like fresh grass, bananas and apples. Hay, cardboard, vinegar, and mud are some of the aromas that indicate an olive oil gone bad."[1]

The idea is to help preserve this incredible delicacy and keep olive oil's vital compounds alive and wholesome. The colour of good olive oil is typically green, or at least that's the way I was taught. Lastly, if you are producing good quality olive oil, you will always provide it in a tinted glass bottle so that damaging sunlight light will be shielded away from the precious product, which you are about to enjoy and sell.[2] In that order of course.

Cooking with oils is a tricky topic as there are a growing number of people who are against both the cooking and consumption of any oil. I've chosen to stay away from that rather purist way of thinking and simply take a stand with reducing heat and being mindful of the susceptibility of oxidation. For the most part, looking at the smoke point is a good idea. Oils that have higher smoke points are generally more resistant to heat. Olive oil sits in the medium category and anyone who cooks will know that it doesn't take very long for the whole kitchen to smell of burnt oil if they aren't cognizant of their stovetop's heat level.

Butter, although smells unbelievably delicious when heated, burns very easily. Just have a look at your cookware on pancake Saturday with the kids and you'll know what I'm referring to. That browned, burnt, butter just isn't as tasty as its raw, unheated predecessor, is it? Then again, applying butter to a warm piece of bread, allowing it to melt ever so softly; now that's a flavour party where everyone's invited. Of course butter is loaded with cholesterol and saturated fat, both of which may not be recommended for someone with high cholesterol or risk of cardiovascular disease. Cooking methods will certainly determine one aspect of fat quality prior to getting absorbed into your system. Do you want to absorb a healthy or unhealthy fat? Oxidized or unoxidized? Seeing how most of us aren't thriving on a solely raw food diet, there are some incredible ways in which you can help preserve your oils as they are being cooked or at least take maximum advantage of the oils. Let me explain.

If you visualize butter in three forms; raw, melted, and browned, there's a noticeable difference in its structure and properties. This holds true no matter what oil you use including motor oil in your car by the way. Some oils just happen to be more resistant to change than others. Sunflower oil, avocado oil, canola oil, grape seed oil, and coconut oil are great examples of plant based oils that have medium to high smoke points which prevent the oil from oxidizing and helps to protect the various health properties contained as well.[3] Regardless, we really shouldn't be cooking using high temperatures, period. After all; it's not only about not eating oxidized oil. More importantly in my view, it's absolutely about taking a leap into the direction of literally choosing to take advantage of many of the healing properties that these oils have to offer. Not cooking these oils, simply mean that these benefits becomes more available for your body to take advantage of.

Young People & Cardiovascular Disease

For the past few decades, we've been under the impression that fat is bad and we should avoid it if we are to reduce risk for cardiovascular disease. Around the 1950's, North America was introduced to mass distribution of fast food and the "American" diet was born. I was astonished to learn about the famous Korean Soldiers Study published in 1955, where the bodies of young, deceased solders of war were studied and what was found was shocking. Early signs of cardiovascular disease in people who were in their ripe late teens to early twenties. [4] Can you believe it? So young. How was this possible? Arterial plaque formation had already begun to form. The following images are from a 1993 follow up study.

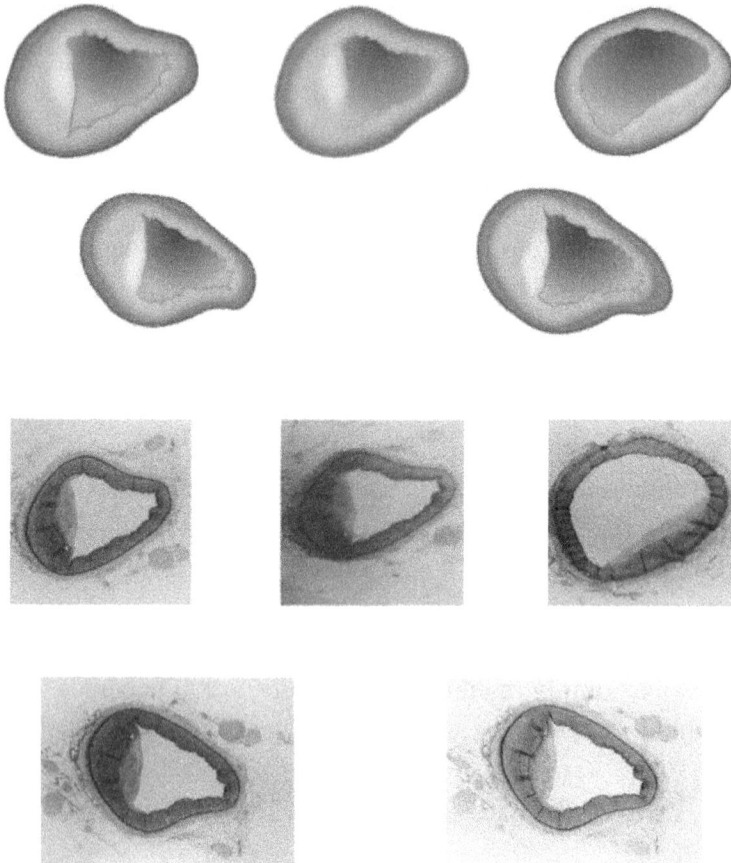

Figure 5: Coronary Atherosclerosis In Young Trauma Victims (recreated in colour) and original (in black and white; Joseph, Abraham et al)[5]

I wonder whether this may be considered as accelerated signs of aging perhaps. Either way, saturated fat was largely to blame as well as high cholesterol, high blood pressure, cigarette smoking, excess weight, elevated blood sugar levels, lack of exercise, stress, and ECG abnormalities. Since then with of course many other examples of high fat diets linked to heart attacks and strokes, the scare continued to escalate and the era of 'low/no fat' foods began.

When I'm reviewing the fat content of someone's weekly diet diary, I'm not simply looking to see how much fat is there so that I say "stop eating fat". No, that would be too easy. Plus, fat is an amazing substance that we can't live without. Even vegetables have some fat. Of course, different kinds and smaller amounts than in a morning Boston Cream donut, but you know what I mean.

I suspect that in order for The Diet Diary to really catch on, it needs a new name. Something ultra-sexy; enticing and motivating even. Any marketing gurus amongst us? 'Medicine's Top Diet Hack - Hint: Results in Just One Week!' I can't stress how important of a tool this can be.

I think we were onto something decades ago. People were certainly increasing their risk of cardiovascular disease, no question. Saturated fat intake may have been a huge link and a fantastic observation, but what we have finally been able to discern a whopping half century later, is that it may not have been merely saturated fat intake.

First off, the shier amounts of saturated fats need to be considered. Next, the lack of other important fats that drive many factors of cardiovascular disease risk need to be given the respect they deserve, including what I along with many believe to be one of the most important risk factors, inflammation. Furthermore, as we saw earlier, when hickory smoked bacon consumption decreased, sugar and carbohydrate intake went up, presumably to bridge that soul satisfying gap.

Needless to say, this trend wasn't in our favour in terms of chronic disease risk.

Vehicles for Oil

The best part of breakfast has to be melted butter with jam on toast in the morning. Still, have you ever attempted pouring olive oil instead, using the bread as a vehicle for incorporating beneficial fatty acids into your diet? Many people assert that I'm crazy for doing it, but I have to ask; when did we get so caught up in having oils become spreadable solids? Salads represent another incredible opportunity for delivering this incredible fat. Plus, there's no need to stop there as avocado and grape seed oil are just waiting to join the party.

Italian cuisine is famous for drizzling room temperature olive oil over readymade food such as pizza. In fact using fine olive oil this way not only tastes better as cooking can change its flavour, but is one of the key factors in the famous Mediterranean Diet, revered for reductions in cardiovascular risk factors such as high cholesterol, high blood pressure, blood sugar intolerances and obesity, coronary heart disease, as well as evidence suggesting possible preventative roles in certain cancers.[6,7] Why succumb to always using grated parmesan cheese over pasta? First off, parmesan is loaded with sodium and high in cholesterol. Can't you just pour over a delicious, high quality olive oil? This not only lends tremendous flavour to the dish but is unbelievably good for you. Pouring room temperature, unheated olive oil over your food ensures that you receive the full benefit of that oil. Where I think most of us shoot ourselves in the foot is the amount that we use as we are using oil twice; during cooking and as a topping, which is certainly a recipe for consuming too many calories, don't you think? Here lies an important opportunity for us to exercise moderation.

Dips have to be one of my absolute favourite ways of incorporating healthy fat simply due to taste and texture. You've probably noticed that hummus has truly taken over shelf space in grocery stores. The ingredients are wholesome and typically few in number, which many of us shoppers equate with healthier, and I'm one of them. With simple ingredients such as chickpeas, garlic, lemon and olive oil, who can go wrong? If you have ever made your own hummus, then you know how incredibly easy it is to prepare, as using even an inexpensive blender can provide enough dip to last a week. Where I see opportunities for improvement, is once again with respect to amount, as most of us simply consume way too much. Whether you make your own or buy at the grocery store, have a look at the calorie and fat content of these dips as you may be surprised. If you're just a little bit careful on the indulgence side of things, you will turn these inexpensive items into some of the healthiest 'supplements' known, right in your very own kitchen, which is truly the best health food store there is.

While creating your masterpiece dip, it is no sweat off your back to include the highest quality, best tasting, health promoting oils of your choice. How do you feel about adding coconut oil to hummus? I know it sounds crazy, but you might actually love it. Grape seed oil offers health benefits with very little taste, whereas olive oil contributes rich, fruity flavours. Sneaking in some avocado may provide a buttery texture that surely won't disappoint. Whatever you try, the key message that I'm attempting to deliver is to incorporate healthy fats, while watching their respective amounts. I believe that was at least one key point we missed decades ago.

One Tool to Rule Them All

There's a simple solution to it all, involving one of the most important tools that health professionals use regularly. A measuring spoon. At first I thought it was a ridiculous idea because I love eye balling my ingredients. Laziness, right? Maybe not just laziness, but perhaps pride. I want to feel as though I somewhat know what I'm doing in the kitchen. Eye balling it seems to give that 'grandmother' feel to cooking. Oh stop it, you know what I mean. Measuring your oil gives you more control. The more I think about it, the more I understand just how ridiculous it is, pouring oil onto a pan straight from the bottle. Why would anyone do that, when you can simply measure the amount of oil with a spoon? I always seemed to have this idea that I needed to literally cover the pan with oil so that food doesn't stick or burn. Of course that shouldn't really happen if you're using non-stick, though not everyone loves the idea.

My wife's grandmother uses iron pots and pans and she's not alone. Many have used this type of cookware for generations. They are incredibly resilient and people swear that they only get better with time. They sort of buildup flavour profiles from various foods over the years. Personally, I don't know how appetizing that sounds, but who am I to argue with a grandmother? As alternatives, stores today are flooded with non-stick cookware that offer huge promise but aren't fool proof as many non-stick surfaces contain chemical compounds that are undesirable for human health, to say the least.

Stainless steel pans don't really have this problem but just like rot iron, food really tends to stick and from personal experience, you need to use a lot of oil. I was living in student residence when I had the bright idea to buy stainless steel. I love the way they feel, as if you're a real chef with some high quality cookware, you know? Washing them afterwards however took a considerable amount of time. My wife advised me to boil water and pour it over, allowing the pan to soak for a while. In all honesty, she lost me at "boil water", let alone "a while".

Ceramic provides an interesting solution which is worth looking into. Non-stick coatings on most home cookware in North America contain perfluorooctanoic acid (PFOA) and other perfluorinated compounds (PFCs), and have been linked to very serious illnesses, which certain ceramic cookware vow to be free of[8]. Besides laboratory findings of reproductive, developmental, and systemic toxicity in animals, these chemicals are bioaccumulating in wildlife and have been found not only in animals but humans too.[9] By having a slippery surface, ceramic cookware naturally requires little oil. Either way, measuring the amount of oil in use, is a great habit to get used to.

If you measure out a tablespoon and it's enough to cook up a meal that serves four people, then it's really only 30kcal of oil per person, which is incredibly reasonable. Therefore, using a measuring spoon before pouring oil will give you a better idea of not only caloric intake but also allow you to ration some calories of oil for cooking and most importantly, poured over top raw once the meal is prepared.

Chapter 10:

Musician or The Band:

The Natural Health Industry's Best Kept Secrets

S ummer is by far my favourite time of the year. I love the heat, and try to appreciate it as much as I can especially considering how long and cold winters here in Canada are. Anyone who knows me understands that there isn't a sole anywhere who doesn't like winter as much as I do. I believe in positivity and 'being the change', don't get me wrong, but everyone has their kryptonite and mine is certainly the bitter cold from January until the end of March. Oh those minus 25 degree Celsius chills. That said, more recently I've attempted to demonstrate at least some sign of maturity, allowing Autumn into my heart.

Being a fan of warm cups of coffee on crisp days, I have certainly come to appreciate the leaves changing colour but more importantly look forward to the food. Fall is probably the very best time of the year for soups, stews, and chilli, all of which are vehicles for flavour and health promoting ingredients. Beans are rich in fibre and protein. Cilantro adds freshness, and colourful chillies give some heat. Rich soup broths are great for the immune system and nourishing for the soul, as they warm the heart. Carefully chosen aromas from spices are also incredibly flavourful and protective, as they encompass some of the most anti-oxidant rich foods on the planet.

I was surprised to learn just how healthy spices are for human health and disease prevention. While cultures all over the world use spices in balance, we seem to be lacking here in the North American diet. One of the most healing spices in the world is without a doubt, turmeric. If you haven't had the pleasure of adding this wonderful herb to your dishes, you're missing out, big time. Human beings have been consuming turmeric for thousands of years and it's incredible that only now, are we finally beginning to understand but a fraction of its medicinal potential. From its anti-inflammatory and antioxidant properties, to diabetes and cardiovascular disease, depression, infection, to digestive concerns and even incredibly protective effects on the liver and anti-cancer research, turmeric is a wonder herb, to say the least.[1] Chances are, you've already been inundated with joint care/pain relief ads for herbal formulas containing this incredible culinary beauty, and I suspect this is just the beginning.

Most turmeric formulas on the market typically don't even really use turmeric at all. They use a tiny fraction of what turmeric represents but market it as a super potent form of its former self. You may see the word "standardized" written on many formulas. Typically, when you grow turmeric in your garden, each plant contains a different amount of what scientists think are the active compounds. That is, what they think are the most useful for therapeutic benefits.

Curcumin is one of turmeric's many incredibly active compounds. Since every turmeric rhizome picked out of the ground, inevitably contains different amounts of this compound, the natural health industry thought there had to be a way to standardize the process so that the public could acquire a consistent dose in every capsule, softgel, liquid, etc. This notion would allow 'good' companies to stand out compared to not so good ones in terms of quality control.[2] In other words, whether you took the first pill or last pill, whether one bottle or your next, you would always be guaranteed to get the same amount of curcumin to help with joint pain, or as an anti-oxidant or whatever it was that you were taking it for. That notion however did not come without a price.

Science is a funny thing. While it is obsessed with pursuing the truth and creating better standards of quality assurance, in terms of the medical industry, I found it to be incredibly reductionistic in its thinking. Everyone's looking for that one single pill that will change everything. The one molecule that will say be the perfect anti-inflammatory or anti-viral, etc. When in reality, time and time again research finds fault in this way of thinking. The truth at least as I see it, is that plants and human beings alike, are far more complicated than any one molecule can ever be. Synergy proves over and over that the whole is greater than the sum of its parts.

Imagine that you and I started a band and I was the best guitarist on the planet and you were the absolute best drummer, and we had the best singer and base player, and so forth. Together we made up one of the greatest bands of all time. The minute that we break up and go off on our own, it's likely that each of us would still produce incredible music, but it's safe to say that the sound that we once created would never be the same again, wouldn't it? This is sort of how I view herbs and medicine to a large degree. While isolated compounds have their place and can certainly accomplish incredible wonders in the body, they lack their full potential but also safety when separated from their original whole. Since there are virtually unlimited amounts of so called active compounds out there, is our mission to ensure that no 'stone goes unturned'? I fear we might be misunderstanding the clues that nature is providing us.

L-arginine can cause blood vessels to dilate.[3] Quercetin[4] and vitamin C [5] have demonstrated anti-histamine properties. Coenzyme Q10 can prevent lipid peroxidation and protect cell membranes against oxidative damage.[6] All of this is interesting, but when placed in the context of whole food, these substances can do so much more and have incredible safety. Everyone knows what will happen if you eat an orange. Conversely, vitamin C (ascorbic acid) can surely be taken at extremely high dosages without exerting much negative effect except probably diarrhea, but by the same token, studies of people taking high dosages of this single nutrient for a long period of time, have shown detriment. In fact, a 2004 study revealed supplemental vitamin C may increase cardiovascular disease risk in postmenopausal women with diabetes. [7] The same goes for vitamin E as although preliminary research was promising, there has been lack of evidence to support long term use. Moreover, taking isolated vitamin E over long periods of time has been correlated with an increased risk of heart disease among both men and women who were either at high risk, or were previously diagnosed with heart disease altogether.[8]

Vitamin C is, well; you might want to sit down for this. Vitamin C in most cases is derived by monstrous levels of processing and chemicals, and is usually isolated from either manipulating glucose [9] or genetically modified corn and tobacco, via a key gene called dehydroascorbate reductase. The increase in this gene of 100-fold could produce up to a 4-fold increase in ascorbic acid[10]. More recent patents involve yeast as an option for less chemical involvement. My question to you is that even without the processing, are we really that desperate to consume copious amounts of an isolated substance? Isn't that more like a drug, rather than a food? I mean; make no mistake, vitamin C is not a food. Vitamin C is a chemical. You may even notice that when you walk into your local health food store, that there are whole food options nowadays. Some of the really knowledgeable staff will often point you in their directions, though not easy, as confused consumers arrive insisting on their 'normal' vitamin C supplement or brand. When comparing price differences between whole food and USP isolates (as they are called: United States Pharmacopeia or USP), it's easy to become confused and go with the less expensive option, especially if you are convinced that they're all the same. That's where a little experience can go a long way.

Turmeric is no different. The level of processing that this wonder herb goes through in order for companies to dig deep and rip out some sort of compound that some scientists believe may be the most active compound at doing some function, is mad science in my opinion. We have literally, as a profession, industry, and consumers alike, convinced ourselves that this way of looking at herbs and food, is the correct way to view their medical offerings. As I mentioned before, there is a large cost associated with this method of naturopathy. Holism and synergy is the way mother nature has always intended and I'll stick with her every time.

When attempting to rip curcumin out of whole, beautiful turmeric, harsh chemicals are typically but not always required. In most cases they involve acetone, toluene[11], dichloromethane, 1,2-dichlorethane (DCE), methanol, ethanol, isopropanol and light petroleum (hexanes).[12] I learned that turmeric powder was actually tested in 2008 whether it could ameliorate liver and heart toxicity from DCE:

"causes irritation to the respiratory tract, damage to the lung, liver, kidney and death due to cardiac toxicity. DCE has been classified as being probably human carcinogen based on the induction of several tumour types in rats and mice treated by garages and lung papillomas in mice after topical application."[13]

I found it intriguing that turmeric powder was being used to ameliorate some of the damaging effects from this dangerous chemical, yet it was the same chemical that has been used numerous times in the extraction of curcumin from whole turmeric itself. I should point out that the study was based on rats by the way, so we're not even entirely sure that turmeric can help in humans against this chemical anyway. Even if it did work in humans, when we rip out the so called active curcumin, we leave behind other beautiful compounds such as turmerones, curcuminoids, and many more that exist in turmeric as a whole. Once they are gone, what's left to 'ameliorate' us then? Just asking.

I'm not in any way suggesting that some curcumin supplements out there are carcinogens themselves, but when harsh chemicals are used, and they are certainly in the majority of cases of standardized herbal extracts (and pharmaceutical drugs too, you might like to know), there is always a residue left behind. Curcumin is awesome in its findings thus far, but it's merely one of over 235 known molecules that make up whole turmeric, and that's what's known so far. This includes primarily phenolic compounds and terpenoids, 22 diarylheptanoids and diarylpentanoids, eight phenylpropene and other phenolic compounds, 68 monoterpenes, 109 sesquiterpenes, five diterpenes, three triterpenoids, four sterols, two alkaloids, and 14 other compounds. Imagine using harsh chemicals to rip out only curcumin and maybe a few other curcuminoids, while sacrificing everything else. Is it worth the risk? Using your own judgement, what do you think the effects are? Of course curcumin is useful in some ways, science has proven that over and over again with literally thousands of published papers, but at the same time, do we truly know what will happen if we take it long term? Turmeric on the other hand, is a herb which we have been taking forever and know innately that as a whole food, we do very well on it.

Absorption Isn't Everything: What Are You Absorbing?

Absorption is highly regarded and sought after within the natural health industry. When walking into a health store only to gaze upon ten 'turmeric' products that sort of looks the same but have different prices attached, often companies will market theirs as being the best, judged according to their self-proclaimed absorption level. In my opinion, this is not the best way of measuring quality, as absorption isn't the most important attribute; not by a long shot. I prefer asking the question, what are you absorbing? If you're absorbing one molecule from one product, a little bit better than that of another, are you truly acquiring something that is more complex? Let's say as an example that you buy two brands of vitamin C and they contain the same amount per pill, at 500mg. One brand absorbs 50% more than the other brand and of course is more expensive. Is it truly a better product? I've asked this question by the way to hundreds of staff within stores all over Canada and many answer yes at first or even perhaps feel as though it's a trick question. I assure you, it's no trick.

I position it like this. I ask them what a really generous dose of vitamin C is. For the record, 60mg is the recommended daily allowance (RDA) to prevent a vitamin C deficiency. Many feel however that our bodies can use much higher dosages to promote optimal health rather than just a pure deficiency and I say "fair enough". I think we can all agree that 5000mg is a huge oral dosage of vitamin C (intravenous aside). At 500mg per tablet (which is pretty average) it means 10 pills, which is a lot, wouldn't you agree? In the higher absorbing brand, they are essentially marketing themselves as being the same value as 7500mg of their competitor, does that make sense? Or in one cases you may be able to take less pills than the other to achieve the same results. Either way, I prefer to look at it differently.

I'm asking the question of whether you believe that you are providing your body with something that is truly more complex in one brand over another? I mean; when even 1500mg per day of vitamin C is a tremendously high dose for say a cold or flu, is 7500mg going to offer your body a noticeable amount of healing benefits when compared to the 5,000mg brand? Will it reduce your cold/flu by a certain number of days over the other guy? I bet you not. Then again, there are other measures such as with respect to anti-tumor effect for example. The higher absorbing stuff may affect certain cancer lines better than the lower absorbing stuff, but again studies are conflicting and this once again raises questions of safety in my mind as well. At the end of the day, more than rate of absorption, I recommend that you consider what exactly it is that you're absorbing. A chemical or a food? Which do you prefer? The same line of thinking can be applied to curcumin, among other supplements and herbal formulas.

Burgos-Moro'n, E et al, described some of these concerns in detail with substantial research in their letter to the editor in the International Journal of Cancer.[14] Curcumin has been shown at high concentrations to induce DNA damage and chromosomal alterations both in vitro and vivo and emphasizes the fact that these are the same concentrations that are attributed to providing therapeutic benefit. They go on to remind us that compromise within DNA is a common thread in cancer risk. I'd like to repeat just how well researched this letter is, just in case 'letter' throws you off as a potentially invalid reference. Full text is available and I encourage you to take a look for yourself. The bottom line however is that studies are conflicting.

We know that when curcumin is ripped out of turmeric the absorption rate drops dramatically but what we also know is that when curcumin is combined naturally with other curcuminoids, absorption is naturally enhanced 7 fold or more.[15,16] You see; curcumin's absorption is naturally high in the context of eating whole turmeric but when chemically isolated, absorption plummets. A black pepper extract called piperine remedies this to an extent as well as fat, which is interesting since it's commonly known all over the world that spices and fats enhance absorption and digestibility of nutrients within foods that we eat anyway.[17] In India, people have been consuming whole turmeric this way for thousands of years. The thought occurred to me years back; if certain compounds work better when consumed in a fat, and some fats are incredibly healthy, and many cultures have been mixing fats with herbs and spices since the dawn of time, shouldn't I be giving more consideration to this type of culinary genius? Big, "yes". Therefore, whenever I remember to do so, I add a little bit of turmeric to oil, specifically for oxidative protection, prior to heating.

Like many, one of my favourite things to do when the weather warms up, is barbecue. One of my patients with high cholesterol couldn't get enough. Marbled rib steak and chicken wings were his favourites and he didn't want to give them up, under any circumstance, and I of course can relate. Look, the truth is that when cooking on a flamed grill, much of the oxidized fat sort of drips down below anyway. It's not that I wasn't concerned about his cholesterol intake, but in this case there was another pressing issue that required attention; burnt food.

My wife Nelly grew up with family gatherings at beaches by a lake every summer, often many times, with full days of deliciously prepared appetizers and real, charcoal, flame grilled barbecue. There's no question about it that grilling meats over coal brings an unmistakable taste to the plate that just can't be beat. Still, I wasn't always a fan. The way I saw it, was that the flame was very much uneven and it was extremely difficult not to burn a large portion of the meat. As I'd be picking away at my lamb, I would hear the 'peanut gallery' constantly remind me "that's [burnt] where the flavour is!" Respectfully, I disagree, though I know where they're coming from.

Nelly's father is famous for preparing the meats in advance, driving at least an hour to a specialty butcher and picking up half a lamb; as in literally a whole lamb cut in half. Who knew that there was a better way of buying meat than the plastic sealed, packaged meats found in grocery stores? He lets the butcher know which cuts he prefers, and like magic, it is so. One year I was lucky enough to be included on this ritual and upon bringing the lamb home, the excitement on everyone's faces was priceless. Just thinking about it, I'm a little disappointed that we didn't make the extra effort this last summer out of pure laziness, I'll be honest.

Everyone's a little bit older now, with kids of their own, and well, that's the excuse. Her father's marinade is epic. Although I can't yet replicate it, bay leaf and lots of thinly sliced onions are imperative. Whatever he uses, after marinating for over 24 hours, the meat is tender as can be and tastes absolutely out of this world over a charcoal flame.

It's as if her father knew something before science ever could. Cultures all over the world have simply known it without any supporting literature, until more recently. You see, when cooking meats, particularly burning them, extremely dangerous chemicals, such as heterocyclic amines (or amino-imidazoazaarenes (AIAs) and polycyclic aromatic hydrocarbons are formed, which are known carcinogens.[18] Very scary stuff. However, a true hero to this story, may reside within my father-in-law's legendary, savoury marinade. In fact, research has shown rosemary, thyme, sage, garlic, and brine are capable of reducing some of these compounds by up to 60% in comparison to not using them.[19] Imagine the power of these herbs and spices.

Oregano and ginger have incredible antioxidant capacity. So much so, that some companies have incorporated these herbs simply because of their ability to help preserve freshness of their oil products against developing rancidity. This affords us an excellent diet diary opportunity, being mindful whether herbs and spices are included within oils and marinades prior to cooking. Although heating should be limited as much as possible, incorporating these simple practices may be worthwhile over time. Lastly, if not for heart health and chronic disease side benefits, doing so provides memorable flavours in your food and satisfaction for your soul.

Chapter 11:

My Father Has Always Had a Love of Basketball

"Why do you want to become a doctor?" This is a question that I have spent nearly my entire life attempting to answer. To this day, I have merely arrived at the same conclusion as I did when I was five years old. Anyone who has ever wanted anything with all their heart, has been faced with this. I maintain that my answer has and always will be the same; "because I want to help people". Of course that would not be good enough on my acceptance interview into medical school, my father advised me. "Admissions is very competitive and everyone else will have something more creative to say," he advised. I needed something different and would have the next 20 years or so to figure it out. Although refined slightly, I admit that I haven't done much 'figuring'. Still, more specifically, the exact answer that I gave on the day when I was finally asked one of the most important questions of my professional life, began with; "My father has always had a love of basketball".

Besides his family, which he adores more than anything, my Dad has always had two big love affairs; music and sport. In pondering the latter, I suppose being part of a team in particular has always meant something incredibly dear to him. The idea of a group of people working hard towards one central goal or idea, inspires greatness. Perhaps that is why he and my mother had four sons (perceived by them to be a relatively large family unit). 'As a unit, the family is strong;' a mantra we have always lived by. Although modestly he was never a great athlete, Dad says that he was a good basketball player. During an intense game in his early twenties, a lateral movement gone wrong had sent him into excruciating pain. His knee was red, warm to touch, and swollen as fluid started to build up almost immediately; inflammation. His doctors diagnosed a torn meniscus in one knee. Surgery was inevitable. Although rehab was endured and healing was diligently pursued, the surgery in many ways was far from a success. He was informed by his physician that not only would he not be able to perform lateral movements during sport, but that it is likely he would never be able to run again as he once could and that he should consider basketball as a thing of the past.

I wanted to be a doctor not just to help anyone, but really to help my Dad; notably with respect to improving physical injuries and inflammation. Originally having the intention to pursue orthopaedics, I focused my naturopathic studies in improving mobility and reducing pain in people who say couldn't throw a baseball in the same way they used to without shoulder pain, or those who were at risk of a hip fracture, especially within the senior or 'expert' population, as I like to call them. We all probably know someone who has experienced osteoarthritis, where beautiful hobbies such as gardening, which often bring such joy, becomes frustrating and at times debilitating. Contributions in this area of wellness is desperately needed, I thought.

Physical medicine and acupuncture became natural points of interest for me, as restoring movement is beyond thrilling, which any physiotherapist or chiropractor can attest. However, I found myself falling into a common trap of believing that inflammation is root of all evil and that in order to sustain lifelong wellness, we need to do everything in our power to defeat it. There have been many books and many more articles written on its negative implications. As a result, many strategies to inhibit inflammation have been tried from both a conventional pharmaceutical model as well as from a holistic healing perspective. Anti-inflammatory and Pro-inflammatory foods, diets, tricks, tips, and supplements have emerged with one focus in mind; to seek out and destroy inflammation. Even "cures" for inflammation have been marketed to drive home its dangers and it's easy to understand why.

Everything from cancer to Alzheimer's Disease, to cardiovascular disease, to nerve problems, eye sight implications, weight gain, aging, and many more health problems are associated with inflammation. Why is that? While I didn't (and still don't) have all the answers, I have long pondered on the foundation of what inflammation really is. Why does the body produce it in the first place? Looking back to basic biology, I think that the following definition at www.biology-online.org is quite useful.

"Inflammation may be acute or chronic. It is a result of a cascade of physiologic processes in response to an injurious agent such as microbes, allergens, etc."

Therefore, I suppose I should start off by clearing up that Inflammation is not only related to pain. There is inflammation that we can feel, and that which we cannot feel, such as within our arteries for instance. This in of itself can oxidize or damage potential fat passing through, or simply cause damage to the artery wall itself. It's this type of inflammation that can lead to plaque formation over time and ultimately heart attacks and strokes. It most certainly doesn't stop at cardiovascular disease, as previously mentioned.

Although genetics certainly play a role in diseases such as Early Onset Alzheimer's Disease, I'd like to share with you that inflammation can contribute to risk factors for diseases pretty much across the board. Even cancer and the aging process itself have huge inflammatory components, which we are only beginning to understand. What about weight loss? Although certain dietary fats can allow the body to influence the way inflammation works, fat storage itself can also be inflammatory in nature. Excess body fat typically increases inflammation. [1] Maybe that's a major reason why obesity increases risk factors for developing a wide range of disease pathology. This is absolutely one of the main reasons in my aforementioned opinion that healthy weight management is one of the most important factors in establishing overall good health.

Alzheimer's disease research over the last few decades have largely been focused around a plaque that forms in the brain, leading to dementia and the horror that is the disease. While drug companies have been looking at how to destroy or prevent plaque formation, it's been expressed by many researchers that Alzheimer's Disease (AD) should be viewed and treated similarly to cardiovascular disease; as a disease of inflammation. In a background paper written in 2004 by Tanna Saloni and updated in 2013 by Beatrice Duthey, Ph.D., taken from the World Health Organization's Website, the paper states:

"Despite occasional negative findings from large prospective studies, the accumulated evidence for a causal role for cardiovascular risk factors and cardiovascular disease in the etiology of dementia and Alzheimer disease is very strong. This has led to speculation that atherosclerosis and Alzheimer disease are linked disease processes, with common pathophysiological and etiologic underpinnings (ApoE ε4 polymorphism, hypercholesterolemia, hypertension, hyperhomocysteinemia, diabetes, metabolic syndrome, smoking, systemic inflammation, increased fat intake and obesity)."[2]

In beginning to learn just how complex inflammation really is, I found myself no longer being able to obsess over regenerating my Dad's knee, allowing him back onto the basketball court. I was now fixated on chronic disease.

Inflammation Is Like a Grenade: The Link to Chronic Disease

As a student, I noticed a common trend within chronic disease. That is, inflammation, sugar, and stress. In fact, this entire book is meant to connect these three basic attributes, using cholesterol as a focal point. Inflammation is so incredibly complicated that the further we investigate, it seems, the 'deeper the rabbit hole goes', and the more dumbfounded the scientific community appears. I myself have attempted to write on inflammation numerous times, ultimately giving up, never really achieving clarity. The more I rely on science and my understanding of cellular behaviour, physiology, and biochemistry, the more apparent it becomes that inflammation as a topic, is an encyclopedia in of itself. Let's take a step back and lean on the basics. Inflammation is like a grenade.

Redness, swelling, and heat; these are common attributes of inflammation. Without going into genetic switches, complicated immune proteins, and other mind boggling variables, at the end of the day, I often view inflammation as being analogous to a grenade's explosion. Let's say that you have 10 grenades side by side. I think we can agree that for the most part they are identical, having the same purpose, exploding once their respective triggers are pulled. There are certainly some aspects of the explosion that we can control such as when we pull the trigger, where to place the grenade, etc. However, controlling the explosion itself is nearly impossible. Moreover, each explosion results in completely different consequences even though categorized in the same way.

The fire, shrapnel, types of property damage caused by the explosion, types of physical damage caused by shrapnel. All of these can be categorized, yet the number of possible outcomes generated are seemingly endless, much in the same way that a snowflake, although created by limited ingredients (water, particles) create an infinite number of different shapes, sizes, and textures. We all have inflammation, governed by more or less the same physical principles across the board. That is, we can control certain aspects such as to a large extent, timing, magnitude, and others, however once it occurs and its processes are set in motion, much as with a grenade, the resulting consequences are unpredictable, with infinite possible outcomes in the body. When this happens periodically over a long period of time, I believe it is our body's natural response to each of these outcomes, that ends up paving roads to different chronic disease states. In one person, they may develop cardiovascular disease, in another Alzheimer's, Crohn's, Psoriasis, cancer; you name it. This is why, in my opinion, with pretty much all forms of chronic disease, we end up seeing common trends with sugar (energy metabolism) and stress being two other top guns on my list.

I'm fascinated with nutrition's ability to influence inflammation and ways in which our body responds, in particular, with respect to fat (energy metabolism). It turns out, that when we eat the right types of fats, in the right amounts, and unoxidized (so raw for the most part), they can help our body's inflammation response work better. That is, our body is actually able to use certain fats from our diet in order to up or down regulate inflammation on a need to need basis. Although complicated, this is very important to be mindful of. After all;

cardiovascular disease is a disease of inflammation. In fact, I love what Peter Libby wrote in a 2006 paper, published in the American Journal of Clinical Nutrition, stating:

"The traditional view of atherosclerosis as a lipid storage disease crumbles in the face of extensive and growing evidence that inflammation participates centrally in all stages of this disease, from the initial lesion to the end-stage thrombotic complications."[3]

The paper is very detailed in describing mechanisms and potential explanations as to why lowering cholesterol even with the use of statin drugs, is thought to reduce cardiovascular events such as heart attacks or strokes. Lowering cholesterol itself is in effect anti-inflammatory, and is demonstrated by influencing an inflammatory marker called C-reactive protein (CRP), which your doctor can easily measure. Lowering cholesterol lowers CRP, so even if you are taking statin drugs such as Lipitor or Crestor, CRP should lower as cholesterol production is lowered. Still, there are many other factors that influence inflammation. You should know that lipid lowering is anti-inflammatory as well, so in other words, lowering fat consumption in general. This effect may differ as a whole in obese from non-obese people, however I tend to gravitate in general towards the following position:

Low fat consumption while maintaining a healthy weight, is by far one of the healthiest approaches we can take. Specifically, eating a variety of unoxidized, non-inflamed fats in low amounts, while not replacing them with excess sugars, carbohydrates, and chemicals (e.g. sugar free options such as Sucralose, Aspartame, etc). This is where moderation is truly tested in my opinion as we can always fool ourselves, but as Mom so eloquently insists, "our body never forgets". By realizing the importance of reviewing your week's worth diet diary (or whatever amount of time you choose), you can help your mind remember too.

Chapter 12:

Over Four Hundred Thousand Stamps

My grandmother lived with rheumatoid arthritis (RA) for over thirty years. She loved to laugh and always used to joke that while everyone called the senior years the 'golden years,' she'd laugh, arguing that they're "the pits". "Enjoy your youth," Omama would tell me. She was in pain. As an avid walker, and I mean avid, her quality of life began to decline as her mobility decreased. Simple joys such as walking 30 minutes to a local grocery store became difficult particularly in the brutal, bone chilling, cold winters of Winnipeg, Manitoba, where her and my grandfather lived for about 20 years. An amazing woman, my Omama was. Born in Vienna, Austria, she suffered a lot in her youth. Like many from that generation, the realities of war shattered her universe. The life that once was; forever changed, as their youth was stolen from them.

While never truly getting over her early tragedies, right up into her old age, she shared with me how the sound of running water made her paranoid. She would remind my grandfather to turn off the faucet as she was concerned about wasting water. I'm talking about the kind of wasting, where she was concerned as to whether there would be any water left. After the war, she had nothing to her name and went hungry many times over. She described herself as never truly getting rid of that mindset; that there may not be another meal around the corner. She was the most incredible cook. Oh wow, was she ever. I just miss it so much. Every last bit of it. The aromas. She wasn't only sharp in the kitchen. Omama carried a survival instinct the duration of her life, being grounded and incredibly wit minded. When my mother's father passed when she was a young girl and my uncle was merely three, they were all lost. As a kind of therapy, Omama relied mostly on stamp collecting an enjoyable, calming past time.

Stamp collecting was her passion and when she sadly passed, I counted very roughly well over four hundred thousand stamps. I decided to write that number out just now instead of simply jotting down 400,000 as it seems to hold more weight. Somewhere during the last 10 years of her life, her memory began fading and she was later diagnosed with Alzheimer's Disease. Seth Rogan, comedian/actor, in 2014 spoke in congress in hopes of raising awareness for the disease. In an article featuring his video, Sarah Devitt (a random woman in his Facebook comment feed) wrote a comment which really stood out for me:

"Alzheimer's is not a gentle condition that causes some mild confusion in only the very aged. It strips relatively healthy people of their memory, their personality, their physical capabilities and their dignity in a vicious unstoppable decline. It does not currently merit the research, medication or most importantly support network level of other diseases and places a huge physical, emotional and financial burden on caregivers."

I wonder whether my grandmother may have been carrying around the disease process itself for decades before it showed signs in the brain. Such a smart and 'with it' woman, with incredible drive and full of energy. How could this have happened? Could her rheumatoid arthritis have been part of the overall process, later manifesting itself as AD? I have been wondering this for the past many years, realizing I'm not alone. As recent as 2014, there have been noted associations between pre-existing cardiovascular disease (CVD), increasing risk of rheumatoid arthritis but not osteoarthritis.[1] Did my Omama have pre-existing cardiovascular disease risk prior to experiencing the onset of her rheumatoid symptoms? I'm honestly not sure. I know that in her later years, she developed diabetes, but how long she showed clinical signs of CVD risk, I really don't know.

Osteoarthritis (OA) is primarily due to wear and tear of the joints, whereas rheumatoid arthritis (RA) is more systemic, possibly a result of immune dysfunction, either way relating to inflammation. Pabau, Helen et al., outlines in the aforementioned 2014 study above that if someone who is at risk of CVD and has family history of RA, then RA should be suspected. In other words, it's quite possible that her RA may have been present though not yet manifesting itself as pain or at the level of pain later on experienced. She may have therefore already been at risk for CVD as there is certainly a parallel between both diseases. We may never know for sure.

Could rampant, chronic inflammation have caused one thing, which led to another, in a sequence of events that eventually caused dementia and then finally a devastating stroke? Rheumatoid arthritis is really a disease of the immune system. It's a condition where the inflammatory response goes haywire and attacks the body in different places. What caused inflammation to go wrong in Omama's case? What could my grandmother have done to help her inflammatory response work better? These are some of many questions that haunt me, but I know I'm not alone. When thinking about the reasons for maintaining healthy cholesterol levels for cardiovascular disease risk, I believe it is in everyone's best interest to consider these questions as well.

The Inflammation Paradigm Shift

I sincerely wish that I could tell you, inflammation is bad and that you should be doing everything in your power to stop it; as if that wouldn't be complicated enough. If you and I could create a drug that worked really well at stopping inflammation, wouldn't it be wonderful? Many have attempted this and I can tell you without doubt that the answer is a most unequivocal "no". In fact, this has been done many times. Researchers found an enzyme system called COX which is simply short for cyclooxygenase that is pretty much responsible for controlling inflammation on a cellular level as we know it.[2] COX-1 and COX-2 are notable. Their thinking was; stop COX, stop inflammation.

Conventional NSAID (Non-Steroidal Anti-Inflammatory Drugs) drugs such Aspirin for instance, have relatively high risk for gastrointestinal toxicity and so people can't rely on them as long term solutions. Drug companies thought that a viable alternative would revolutionize treatment of pain related diseases such as arthritis; a noble ambition, no doubt. Rofecoxib (Vioxx), Celecoxib (Celebrex), and Valdecoxib (Bextra) were born as three drugs that do a very good job at this. The problem is that drug companies, although probably having great intentions, didn't realize that inflammation is both good, bad, and ultimately necessary. Previously, it was thought that COX-2, although playing a role in pain, had no bearing on homeostasis or balance, basically. That way of thinking was wrong and was proved unfortunately through serious undesirable side effects, such as cardiovascular toxicity and death.[3] Vioxx and Bextra were taken off the market as quickly as they were brought on. If we learned anything from this, it was that inflammation is complex.

While in the short term, we can certainly use drugs to influence physiology, inflammation is analogous to a vast network that continuously changes, accommodating for different variables. We can't change one aspect without taking the whole picture into consideration. Think about it; we need inflammation to heal, don't we? Inflammation is also an integral part of the immune response. During an infection, we need our immune system to find the pathogen responsible, responding promptly. The finding, fighting, cleaning up, as well as the healing process itself, are all intimately connected with a properly functioning inflammatory response. Thus, it is our duty to understand and appreciate that our mission isn't to stop inflammation as the drug companies would have us believe, but rather it is to help our inflammatory response work the best that it can for as long as it can.

It seems as though despite its importance for survival, every time inflammation occurs, it comes at a small cost. Should we be placing ourselves in a position where we spread out inflammation for as long as possible? Inflammation is a kind of natural medication for the body. In the same way that pharmaceutical drugs can be palliative, certainly taking drugs as infrequent as possible is a good overall strategy. Inflammation is a wonderful 'drug', but does it come with the cost of slowly but surely contributing to chronic disease?

A quick look at any inflammation diagram will surely make you nauseous as they are absolutely daunting. With so many different pathways to consider, researchers scramble to find rate limiting steps so that they can determine which one can be controlled by what substance, and so forth. An example is A turns into B using X, which then using some Y turns into C, and so forth. Below, I have included an easy to read diagram in layman terms, illustrating complexity, followed by a scientific one, describing key component of inflammation for your viewing pleasure involving the arachidonic acid pathway.

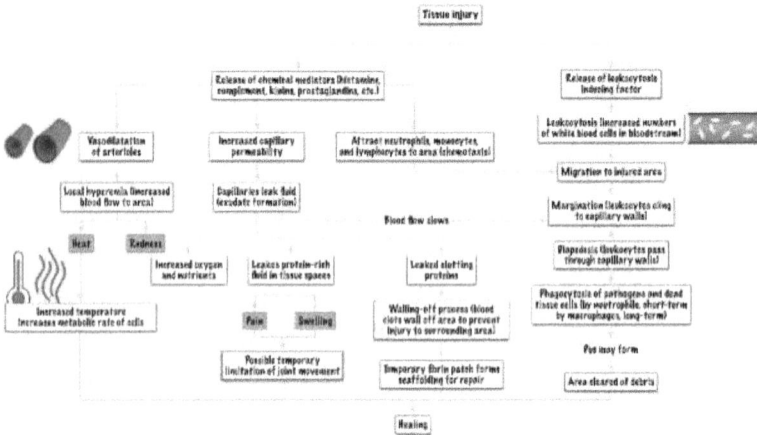

Figure 6: Simple Layman Terms Inflammation (recreated from original; Benjamin Cummings, 2001)[4]

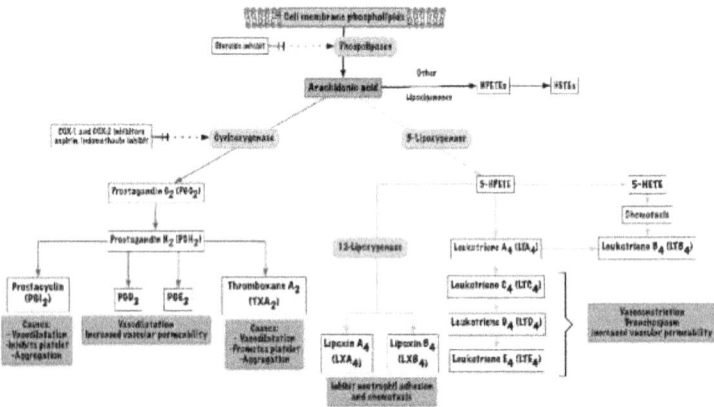

Figure 7: Arachidonic Acid Metabolites an Inflammation.[5]

Would you eat fat as an anti-inflammatory supplement? After reading this, you might start. Fats offer an incredible contribution to our body's ability to regulate inflammation. This is in fact a huge reason for the entire omega-3 campaign.

You've probably seen it everywhere, haven't you? Omega-3 enriched eggs, breads, seeds, snacks, and more; all of which have suddenly been marketed towards educating consumers about their respective essential fatty acid content. In a big way, this is a result of inflammation and heart health. The reason without going into all of the chemistry, can truly be summarized by looking at a variety of fats. Basically, there are many omegas, each with their own amazing contributions but as healthy as these fats can be, moderation but moreover context to which food they are derived, must be taken into consideration in my opinion.

Omega-3 is well known and really one of, if not the best source, is from fish. Olive oil contains omega-9 (oleic acid), which has been studied to confer its own unique benefits with respect to cardiovascular health, including studies showing its ability to lower elevated LDL cholesterol, but extends beyond in many respects from reduction in insulin requirements in type 2 diabetics, to omega-9 enriched LDL cholesterol, conferring more resistance to oxidative stress, as well as immune benefits and properties contributing to vasodilation within arteries, among other.[6] One of the boldest statements that I've seen is that olive oil is considered to be the major antiatherogenic or anti-arterial plaque forming component of the Mediterranean Diet.

Sea buckthorn has become a local favourite amongst some of my colleagues, and if you walk into a local health food stores these days, you may see this ingredient in many ultra-premium skin care lines. One of the many active ingredients of this plant's fruit has created a pretty loud buzz within the natural health industry. Omega-7 (palmitoleic acid) has been implicated in many topical skincare products to treat wounds and burns.[7] Sea buckthorn has been used for over a thousand years in Traditional Chinese Medicine since the Tang Dynasty for diseases of the skin, gastric ulcers, asthma and other lung disorders. While Western medicine is behind, it's surely not in the dark, as recent research has begun accumulating and revealing pharmacological properties such as antioxidants, immunomodulatory, anti-atherogenic, anti-stress, liver protective, protection against radiation, and enhanced tissue repair.

Most vegetable oils such as sunflower contain omega-6. Some foods contain a natural mix of many different fats. In fact, if you look at the label of a wild Pacific salmon oil product, you may notice omega 5, 6, 7, 9 as well as other naturally occurring beneficial compounds. What's fascinating is that salmon actually contains more relative amounts of omega-7 than even sea buckthorn does. Salmon oil is revered for skin health in general as well.

While each of these fats may be unbelievably healthy for human health in moderation, the most important thing that I've ever learned regarding any of them is that none of them is the elixir of life. No single compound found thus far has been found to even closely resemble the fountain of youth. Olive oil of course has its slew of benefits including, but not limited to helping out our nervous and immune system, among others. Coconut oil has its array of uniqueness and there have been many books written about the "miracles" of this natural wonder food. While all of these stories may be compelling, I have found that that the best level understand thus far has come within the guidelines of balance, the exact of which we pretend we know but are truly not even close to fully comprehending.

Omega-3 to omega-6 balance has been the topic of conversation within the natural health industry, particularly over the last decade or so. Laboratory tests have been created to inform people of their specific ratio. Some researchers have postulated that an optimal ratio is 1. In other words, we should be eating about the same amount of omega-6 as omega-3, as this is what human beings are theorized to have eaten in our ancestral past[8]. The North American diet has been found to paint a dramatically different picture as we tend to consume between 15-20 times omega-6 as we do omega 3.[9] Just imagine. This idea started a marketing revolution, where the natural health industry threw omega-6 under the bus for a long time. To this day, some savvy health people question eating anything containing omega-6 because of this fact. When discovering that salmon in addition to being a great source of omega-3, does contain a proportional amount of omega-6, they cringe. It's true, I've witnessed this personally.

Omega-6 is a wonder drug; you just don't know it yet. The body needs omega-6 fatty acids from vegetable oils for many bodily functions, however are over abundant within North American diet, notably within over cooked foods such as French Fries or as my American compadres like to call, 'Freedom Fries'. Whichever way you look at it, potato chips, crackers, stir fries and many other common items surrounding us daily, typically use vegetable oils (omega-6).

North Americans aren't alone, as 'take-out' definitely has more than its fair share. Haven't you noticed the way these foods typically smell? Delicious! No, but seriously, haven't you noticed that burnt smell in many of your favourite noodle dishes? These foods are typically cooked at extremely high temperatures hence the 'fast' in fast food. Omega-6 is so unbelievably necessary in balance with what our body needs, but of course our society goes overboard, consuming it in almost everything and then overheating it. Fried foods which have become a staple in our diets, provide not only excess calories low on the nutrient density totem pole, but moreover some of the most dangerous fat available; oxidized and/or burnt.

The American Heart Association suggests there is benefit when replacing saturated fats with omega-6 polyunsaturated fats, but of course this is all in the context of adequacy.[10] It has been reported that adequate daily intake of these fats carries more weight than picking apart specific ratios. Both omega-3 and omega-6 are unbelievably healthy, just that omega-3 appears to be in a deficient state. The bottom line is to trade in deep fried foods and snacks in boxes, for small or moderate amounts of your finest, healthy, raw, organic sunflower oil (omega-6) instead.

I learn something new about olive oil, almost every single time I read about it. A new health compound seems to pop up, and I become re-inspired. It is as if I have discovered the next best thing that everybody absolutely needs to hear about, every time I pick up a bottle. Imagine any one of the following compounds being the next big supplement on the market; oleuropein, hydroxytyrosol, caffein acid, protocatechuic acid, and 3,4-dihydroxyphenylethanol-elenoilic acid for cardiovascular disease prevention, secoiridoids and lignans for prevention of tumoral disease, hydroxtyrosol and other polyphenolics possessing anti-inflammatory activity, oleuropein with antimicrobial and antiviral properties.[11] Of course innately, we know that olive oil cannot be reduced to merely a few compounds, and by the way when I say a few, I really mean a few hundred probably. Eating whole, rich, minimally processed olive oil, feeds into what we have been doing for millennia so besides the health benefits, there is a vast confidence level in safety. When we start isolating interesting molecules or 'active compounds' out, and introducing them into our blood stream, there is truly no telling what they will do, regardless of short term, 'fad research', especially where chronic disease is concerned. I believe that same concept can be applied to whole foods.

When we eat a wide variety of whole foods, there is a synergy there. What will happen if a person sticks to eating one food their entire life? In fact, when I think of our beloved animal family members, why are we feeding dogs and cats pretty much the same foods day in and day out? Does that seem healthy? The same concept is what I apply to healthy fats when looking at a person's diet diary. I specifically look for both amounts as well as variety of healthy, minimally processed/cooked oils, as that is truly what I believe will bring about the greatest positive impact on cardiovascular disease prevention and quite possibly, chronic disease prevention in the broader sense.

Having omega-6 in balance with omega-3, reduces inflammation. This is a sentence that is not entirely accurate in my opinion. I don't think it's fair to simply say that foods are pro or anti-inflammatory in nature, as the body doesn't work that way. I'd rather look at it in terms of balanced omega fatty acids help the body to determine whether it needs more or less inflammation. Maybe when we introduce oxidized fat, the body simply needs inflammation as the immune system identifies it as being foreign and not appropriate for human consumption. Many think about it as what fat can do to our body. I believe it's more of what are bodies can do with fat.

If you're taking B-vitamins for energy, consider perhaps that these vitamins aren't what you think they are. In fact, B-vitamins are really just chemicals, having no caloric value whatsoever. So, energy they are not. I'd rather state it like this; your body can use these chemicals to produce energy, depending on what state you are in, and what you need in order to perform whatever task you are trying to accomplish. If you're physically active for example and your metabolism is converting fat to produce energy for muscles to function, then you will certainly use b-vitamins in converting sugar into usable energy within your cells. Fats act in the same way. Your body is so incredibly complex that it will use a large variety of fats to help perform better, depending. Having a variety is certainly key.

The following four figures show how we are able to control biochemical pathways towards building more or less inflammation, according to need via omega-3 and omega-6 fatty acid intake, as well as a non-exhaustive list of inflammatory diseases and conditions whereby marine omega 3 fatty acids may be beneficial.

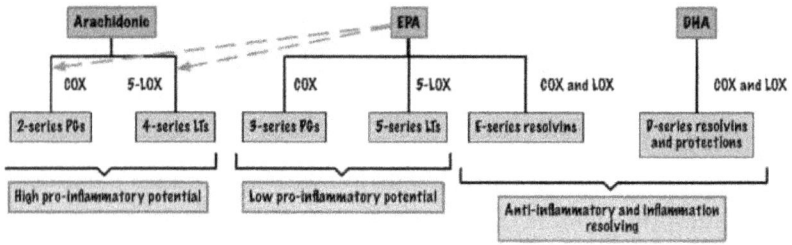

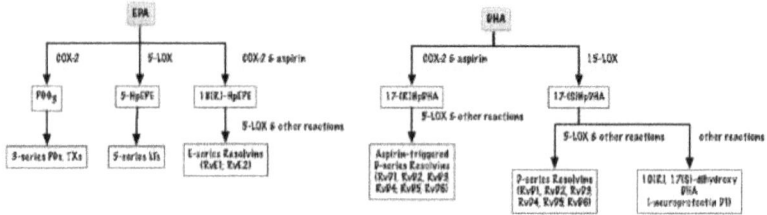

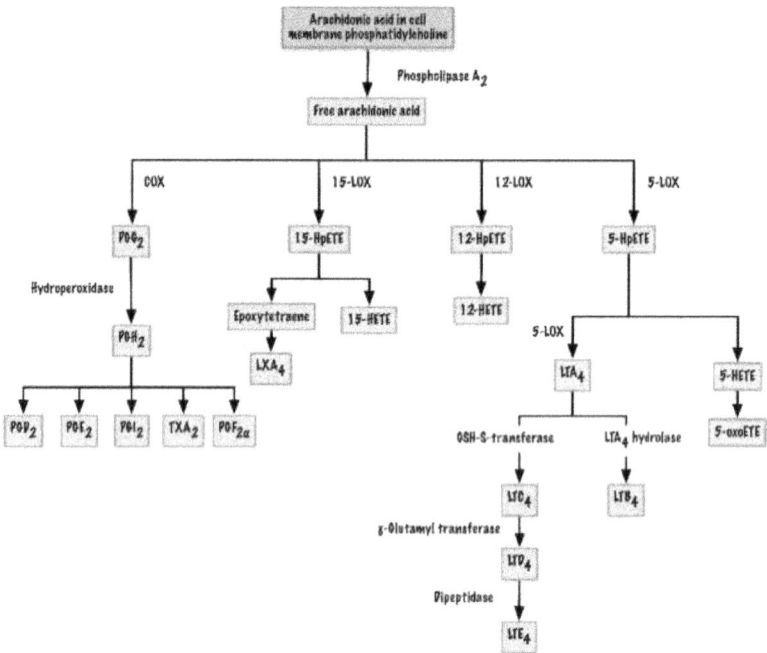

Disease/condition
Rheumatoid arthritis
Crohn's desease
Ulcerative colitis
Lupus
Type-1 diabetes
Cystic fibrosis
Childhood asthma
Adult asthma
Allergic disease
Chronic obstructive pulmonary disease
Psoasis
Multiple sclerosis
Atherosclerosis
Acute cardiovascular events
Obesity
Neurodegenerative diseases of aging
Systemic inflammatory response to surgery, trauma and critical illness

Figure 8: Biochemical (omega-3 and omega-6 fatty acids) pathways towards building more or less Inflammation[12]

Arachidonic acid promotes inflammation and although modest amounts of omega-6 keeps it at bay, too much will achieve the opposite. In my opinion, adding omega-3 supplements to your regimen will not really bring 'balance'. Don't get me wrong, you might observe positive changes in your omega-6 to omega-3 ratio, but what about your other fatty acids; should you try and create 'perfect ratios' for each of those too, using supplements? Maybe you'd like to achieve the perfect ratio of nutrients as well. That's not only cumbersome in thought, but impractical in nature. I'm going to share with you what I think is our best current strategy to sway balance in our favour, using enough of a variety of whole, delicious, nutrient dense foods, to help you function as optimally as you can, for as long as you can, promoting lifelong wellness.

Chapter 13:

How Do You Like Your Eggs?

Eggs, butter, and coconut oil, are amongst the most debated items regarding cholesterol health. It's not too difficult to understand I suppose, as we just love them so much. Who doesn't look forward to eggs, especially on Saturday when Dad's finally home cooking, right? I know I'm being a little backwards thinking here. For one thing, some of the best chefs in the world are men. For another, mom's work just as hard if not harder than us gents, but stay with me here. While my three younger brothers and I were growing up in the 80's and 90's, moms were still living up to some hefty expectations.

Women in North America were acknowledged and respected in the work force, yet the title of Home Maker still lingered as an assumption. The tasks of bringing home 'equal rights bacon', cook and clean, and still act as Doctor Mom and Super Mom in their 'spare time' were not easy. Mom prepared incredible, healthy meals all the time when we were kids. Yet as delicious as they were, we looked forward to Dad's simple meals, early Saturday mornings.

Salami omelet is his specialty. Step 1: place salami on hot pan without adding oil, as there are already beautiful, white fat globules naturally occurring within the meat. As the pan heats up, they effortlessly melt together, providing an aroma that initiates one satisfying morning. Step 2: crack whole eggs into a bowl and whip vigorously. Step 3: add a pinch of salt and pepper; you know the drill. Only once the salami is super crisp, will Dad pour over the eggs. Once everything is cooked evenly, a magical flip, and ba-baam! Oh wait, I forgot the best part.

As a coffee man, he couldn't possibly leave his kids behind, could he? Four chocolate milks, coming right up! Not hot chocolate. Cold, chocolate milk, using Nestlé® Quick powder. Breakfast of champions. On the morning of my wedding day, I awoke only to find Dad already 'up and at em', mastering the omelet of my dreams. Absolutely nothing like it.

Chocolate milk; I get it. The sugar, chemicals, and even a full glass of milk is debatably not the healthiest thing in the world. I say debatable because thousands, if not tens of thousands of publications, both support and oppose human consumption. Momentarily, I will explore some key findings differentiating organic from non-organic. Nevertheless, lets label milk as neutral in moderation, and call it a day.

Salami is of course incredibly unhealthy. Saturated fat and sodium content are through the roof. Cold cuts in general undergo a tremendous amount of processing and include dangerous additives. Nitrates are linked with horrible consequences to human health, if consumed over long periods of time. Yet, the United States Environmental Protection Agency indecisively wrote in their 2007 TEACH Chemical summary (Toxicity and Exposure Assessment for Children's Health):

"Exposure to higher levels of nitrates or nitrites has been associated with increased incidence of cancer in adults, and possible increased incidence of brain tumors, leukemia, and nasopharyngeal (nose and throat) tumors in children in some studies but not others. The U.S. EPA concluded that there was conflicting evidence in the literature as to whether exposures to nitrate or nitrites are associated with cancer in adults and in children."[1]

Intuitively, both nitrates and nitrites (a metabolite from nitrates) seem unhealthy. However, curing meats and poultry has been a practice for over 5000 years. Nitrites prevent fats and oils from going rancid and causing harm. Some research actually shows that nitrite has antibacterial effects on fish muscle, even botulism causing bacteria that used to be relatively large problems from sausages, meats.[2] For a long time, the majority of research focused on vegetable sources, which is why harmful effects have been difficult to find. Vasodilation, as a result of increased nitric oxide production, confers a host of side benefits alone. It wasn't until refrigeration was introduced for prolonging shelf life in meats and other foods, did we investigate further.[3] In the 1970's, carcinogenic compounds created from sodium nitrite, called nitrosamines, initiated the debate.

In 2009, there was an astonishing paper published in the Journal of Alzheimer's Disease (AD), which connected nitrosamine to AD, Type 2 Diabetes Mellitus (T2DM) and Non-Alcoholic Steatohepatitis (fatty liver disease). [4] Researchers describe mechanisms by which nitrosamines cause DNA damage via mutations, resulting in inflammation, oxidative stress, and breakdown in cellular repair machineries. Here is an excerpt from the study:

"Nitrosamines exert their toxic and mutagenic effects by alkylating N-7 of guanine, leading to increased DNA damage [8], and generation of reactive oxygen species such as superoxide (O_2-) and hydrogen peroxide (H_2O_2), which result in increased lipid peroxidation, protein adduct formation, and pro-inflammatory cytokine activation [9]. However, these very same molecular and biochemical pathogenic cascades are associated with major human insulin- resistance diseases, including Type 2 Diabetes Mellitis, Non-alcoholic steatohepatitis, and Alzheimer's Disease. [10–16]. The concept that chronic injury caused by exposure to alkylating agents could result in malignancy and/or tissue degeneration is not far-fetched … Therefore, although research on nitrosamine-related compounds has been largely focused on their mutagenic properties, thorough characterization of their non-neoplastic and degenerative effects is clearly warranted."

The conclusion of this study is so powerful that I am compelled to share:

"In conclusion, environmental and food contaminant exposures to nitrosamines play critical roles in the pathogenesis of major insulin resistance diseases including Type 2 Diabetes Mellitis, Non-alcoholic steatohepatitis, and Alzheimer's Disease. Improved detection and prevention of human exposures to nitrosamines will lead to earlier treatments and eventual quelling of these costly and devastating epidemics."

Below is a chart showing preservative containing meats in Australia (just for the heck of it):

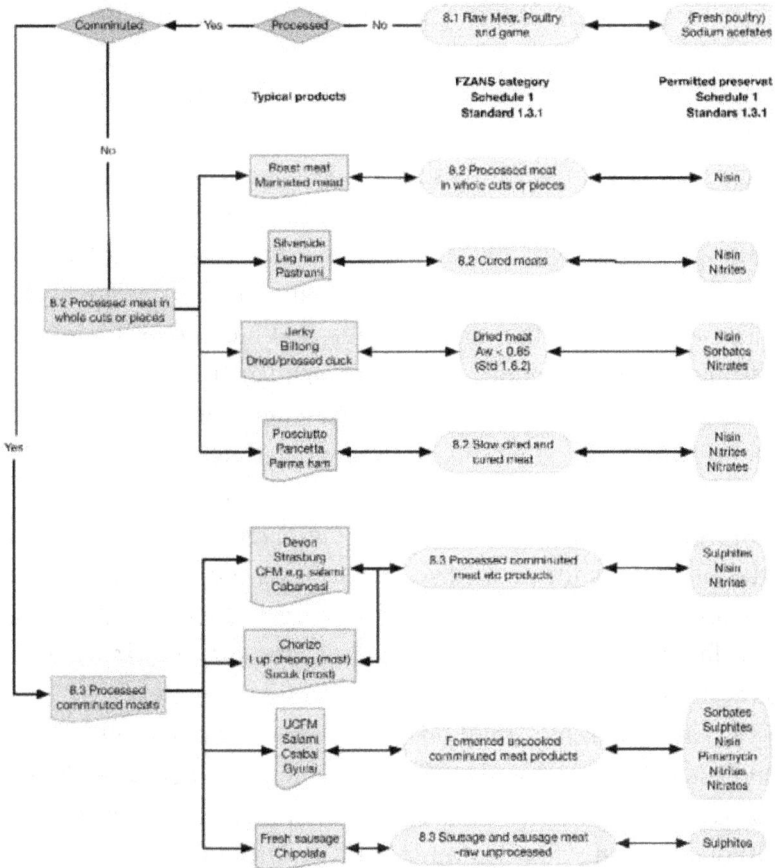

Figure 9: Preservative containing meats in Australia (recreated from original)[5]

Cold cuts are not healthy protein sources. As a result, Mom rarely allowed them. You could say that they were almost an endangered species at home. Still, Dad always managed a special reserve. Nowadays, I can sleep through a lion's roar, but there is nothing like waking to the smell of Dad's breakfast right before Saturday morning cartoons.

93% Of Daily Cholesterol in One Egg

Eggs are loaded with cholesterol. The heart and stroke foundation recommends 200mg per day for someone with increased risk of cardiovascular disease and up to 300mg per day otherwise.[6] Consider this; one large egg contains about 186mg. 2 eggs will place you above the recommended daily maximum even if you aren't at high risk for cardiovascular disease. So what's the deal with eggs? What happens when you eat that 3 egg omelette? The short answer, is that we have no idea. Eating a massive 3-4 egg omelette every once in a blue moon won't do anything to you as far as anyone can tell, except grant you enormous amounts of awesome nutrition. Oxidized, inflamed, or basically 'damaged' cholesterol, is the true risk factor for heart disease as far as our best, most recent research eludes.[7,8,9] When it comes to eggs, therefore the largest risk factor is really a combination of amount, cooking method, as well as internal inflammation and oxidative stress.

I say "cooking method", as heat unfavourably change cholesterol within an egg. The yolk changes when scrambled or as part of an omelet. Conversely, over-easy or sunny side up, although warm, for the most part is left unharmed, thus the overall healthier cooking methods. Yes, poached works as well. My wife refers these preparations simply as "eggs dip". I always manage to over-cook at least one of hers, despite mine turning out perfect. Buttered toast with strawberry jam, dipped in warm, liquid egg yolk? Salivating.

I say "amount" of eggs, as even unharmed cholesterol, can still pose a cardiovascular threat. Inflammation and oxidative stress exists within our arteries despite not being able to physically feel it. I believe we need to evaluate both the shier amount of cholesterol as well as cooking method. More comprehensively, promoting a healthy inflammatory and stress response, and energy metabolism. We are constantly bombarded by forces of nature, which demand inflammation and oxidation for protection and preservation of life. The oxygen paradox is a great reminder of how dependant we are on breathing, yet how deleterious it is to our health and the aging process.[10] Dr. Aubrey de Grey mentioned in his recorded transcript from The Future of Health Now 2012:

"It's the chemistry of breathing – the chemical combination of oxygen with nutrients to create carbon dioxide, of course, but also to release energy from our nutrients – that process is the main way by which our body produces free radicals, which are of course toxic chemicals that can damage our DNA and our proteins in other parts of the body. And that is certainly a large part of why we age. So we're not going to be able to stop that from happening, and that means we have to figure out other ways to remove that damage before it accumulates to a level that causes us problems."[11]

The reason why antioxidants don't work, he explains, is because our metabolism, although generates free radicals that are toxic, also requires free radicals to survive. If by some miracle antioxidant supplements could eliminate oxidation in our bodies, they would kill us by the same token. It's a matter then of helping our own body's natural mechanisms work better. Regarding cholesterol and triglycerides, cooking method and amount can sway in our favour.

Chapter 14:

No Sushi, Chinese, Or Thai Food

You know, the more that I talk about food, the more I truly don't understand why my Dad doesn't cook more often. He's not alone. Many people just don't have a taste for it. My wife insists that she falls in the same category, yet she's an incredible cook. For me, preparing my own food comes down to survival, passion, and control. Author Michael Pollan, describes these attributes perfectly in his book Cooked: A Natural History of Transformation. [1] It's a magnificently written book, where he takes great care in describing what cooking means, not only to him, but to the human race. The act of cooking, he points out, is a basic foundation of survival, which we must carry forward. Otherwise we risk losing a piece of our history going back to the dawn of fire.

We have become a society that relies mostly on the work of experts in various fields. An expert in farming is relied upon by most of us who don't have the ability, the time, or the passion to grow our own food. Yet, we laypeople often distrust the food we eat, don't we? Chemical fertilizers, pesticides and herbicides, and GMOs, are hot topics, which have contributed to huge paradigm shifts in consumer buying trends, towards labeling items with third party certifications. Growing our own food, would change that.

Ok fine, I'm a realist. I don't want to grow my own food. Mostly, because I'm deathly afraid of bees. I highly respect them, so please 'bee' nice. Unequivocally there is nothing like picking a fresh apple right off a chemical-free tree, or pulling off some fresh basil leaves and crushing them into a bowl of soup or tomato sauce. Still, most of us aren't willing to turn our land into farm land.

With many families being supported by dual income, it's not so easy to find time to cook. Plus, who doesn't love going out to eat? Food is prepared by experts, there's no cleanup to concern yourself with, and ultimately, the reward at the end of a long hard day at the office seems more than worth it. Be that as it may, something intimate has most certainly been lost, Michael Pollan, elaborates. After all; there is something truly remarkable about the act of preparing a meal from start to finish, using fresh ingredients, while gathering as a family unit. Furthermore, having a certain level of appreciation for where our food is grown to how it's prepared, increases conscious awareness of what we are putting into our bodies.

Having two of the best kids this green Earth has ever seen, I admit that my wife and I don't go out nearly as much as we used to. If you have kids, you know exactly what bringing them to a restaurant entails. It's disruptive to say the least. Babies as I've discovered, are the easy ones. 'Milk drunk' is a term that I've familiarized myself with and equate it with an adult 'food coma' following a large, satisfying meal. The 2 year olds, are far more challenging to say the least.

Bringing a screaming, jumping, frustrated two-year-old to a restaurant full of hard working people who just want to have a quiet night out, is not a good idea. If you have children, grandchildren, nieces, or nephews, I know what you're thinking. You didn't have those issues with yours as they were far better behaved than that. Well, I'm here to tell you, "No. No they weren't". For these and countless other reasons, take-out is often the right 'sugar to help the medicine go down'.

Some of the best naturopathic medical knowledge I've received, is from my mom. "You're a naturopathic doctor and you need to set an example. No more sushi, Chinese food, Thai food." Story of my life. She's right of course. Funny enough, whenever I'm surrounding by colleagues who are either practising in clinics or working within the natural health industry, Thai, Chinese, or Sushi always seem to be the foods of choice.

Chinese Food, or at least the more commonly found take out stuff, is an easy one to figure out. Deep fried, fatty meats, very high cooking temperatures, massive amounts of calories, and MSG (monosodium glutamate), and that's just the beginning. Some of my favourite teenage memories include sitting outside on a curb, eating local, Chinese take-out. Taste-wise, there's nothing like crispy, crunchy, deep fried wontons with extra sweet and sour sauce for dipping. As far as health is concerned, inexpensive inflammation and oxidative damage in a bag, is more like it.

Sushi is confusing. On one hand, you should receive praise for incorporating omega-3 rich salmon into your diet. In fact, salmon contains over 17 known omega fatty acids, in balance, as nature intends. Moreover, salmon is a great natural source of both astaxanthin and vitamin D3. Finally, those proteinaceous, thirty pieces of raw sashimi, will certainly be used for building muscle tissue from last night's workout. Credit here is due.

New sushi places are opening up around every corner and fish is uniquely consumed raw. Thus, parasitic contamination is more likely. Sourcing is also questionable, however in fairness, all grocery stores and seafood restaurants alike should be critiqued. Farmed fish in general, contains pesticides as well as harmful, industrial, chemicals called polychlorinated biphenyl (PCBs) and dioxins. These are classified as persistent environmental toxins, which are neurotoxic, carcinogenic, act as endocrine disrupters.[2,3] Most of the farmed salmon being distributed in the U.S. originates from Canada and Chile. As a Canadian myself, I was appalled to learn that farmed salmon from Canada, Maine, and Norway have been tested for double the contaminants as those from Washington State and Chile. Dioxin-like compounds and cancer risk are so pronounced, that a collaborative research article featured in Environmental Health Perspectives in 2005 wrote:

"Only wild Pacific salmon can be consumed at rates of ≥ 4 meals/month (1 meal/week), with consumption rates for the least contaminated wild salmon > 16 meals/month (4 meals/week) .... to achieve a cancer risk of 1×10^{-5} (the middle of the U.S. EPA's acceptable risk range; U.S. EPA 2000), consumption of [most] farmed Atlantic salmon must be effectively eliminated and consumption of wild salmon must be restricted generally to less than one meal per month."[4]

Pickled ginger and green tea are among healthier options at a sushi all you can eat menu. Yet, how focused and driven do you really feel immediately following your epic meal, from these ingredients? I thought so. Also, massive amounts of sticky, white rice will inevitably raise your triglycerides, which is counterproductive for someone with high cholesterol or increased risk of cardiovascular disease.[5] To top it off, many of the other menu items are deep fried, such as tempura or those flattened, old, frozen, deep fried 'scallops'. Soy sauce is high in sodium and even the 'low' kind will have you drinking water at the office like a fish for the rest of the day. The creamy mayonnaise contained within many items combined with sugary sauces, place sushi not far behind Chinese food in my opinion.

Thai food is my take-out food of choice, which places me in a bad position. My wife absolutely hates the taste of coconut, yet she loves sharing food. There are very few instances where I eat anything containing it. Turning down Thai food is not easy for me. I'm not a powerful man, yet feed me a plate full of Massaman curry and time stands still. Sweet, creamy, and just the right level of spice. While inhaling the meat and vegetables, drenched in a nutty, coconut milk curry, I'm in heaven. The more I eat, the more I want.

Nowadays there are exciting, new, certified organic coconut products popping up everywhere. After all, virtually all parts can be used. Coconut water has become famed for its supremacy for athletic performance enhancement, delivering electrolytes without added sugar, artificial flavouring, or colouring agents. You may also be intrigued to learn that the shell is used in major household water filtration systems. It seems as though the oil is bound by no limits.

Decades ago, my mom as well as the rest of the world, knew coconut oil as a source of saturated fat. As a result, we didn't eat it growing up. Until several years ago, I didn't give it a second thought. It was while working at a very well respected organic, whole food distribution company. They sold certified organic coconut oil before the massive retail explosion occurred, as far as I could tell. I was inspired with new possibilities of what this food can do for human health.

The Oil That Could

Science has been investigating the topical application of coconut oil on skin wounds. It has been postulated that its saturated fatty acid structure, by preventing rancidity longer than say that of olive oil, along with its nutrient density, offers unique healing qualities.[6] A 2010 study performed in rats, revealed improvements along many parameters. Everything from decreased time of complete epithelization, to higher collagen cross-linking, and even increasing antioxidant enzyme activities.[7] This kind of research has been expanded into the field of sun protection, where 20% of harmful ultraviolet rays were blocked.[8] Moreover, coconut oil's moisture, antioxidants, and nutrient content is healthy for skin regardless.[9]

Cooking with coconut oil has become so popular, that huge organic tubs are available in bulk wholesale stores. First, it doesn't burn as easily as olive oil. Second, it's a fantastic energy source, and tastes fantastic. Still, its saturated fat content is a concern, or is it? Since canola oil has a high smoke point, why not choose it instead? You absolutely can. However, if you are the person who truly loves margarine as a spreadable butter replacement, coconut oil, also a solid at room temperature, might just win you over. Here's why.

Oxidized fat and inflammation are some of the true culprits of chronic disease in my opinion. With a medium to high smoke point, coconut oil is advantageous over butter. Furthermore, the type of saturated fat makes a difference. Butter and coconut oil contain long chain and medium chain triglycerides, respectively. As it turns out, medium chain triglycerides are more readily taken up by the body as an energy source instead of being stored as extra fat.[10] We're all familiar with the fact that in countries whereby saturated fat consumption is the highest, so tends to be deaths from heart attacks and strokes, right? Wrong. As it turns out, the complete opposite is true, reported Dr. Conrado S. Dayrit in a 2003 edition of the Philippine Journal of Cardiology. He states:

"The countries consuming the highest amounts of coconut oil – the Polynesians, Indonesians, Sri Lankans, Indians, Filipinos – have not only low serum cholesterol but also low coronary heart disease rates – morbidity and mortality.

The reason why coconut oil cannot be atherogenic is basic. Coconut oil consists predominantly of 65% medium chain fatty acids (MCFA) and MCFAs are metabolized rapidly in the liver to energy and do not participate in the biosynthesis and transport of cholesterol. Coconut oil, in fact, tends to raise the HDL and lower the LDL: HDL ratio. Coconut oil is not deposited in adipose tissues and therefore does not lead to obesity. It is primarily an energy supplier and as fast a supplier of energy as sugar. MCFAs therefore differ in their metabolism from all the long chain fatty acids, whether saturated or unsaturated."

Chapter 15:

A Little Health Food Store University:

Herbal Formulas & Sports Supplements

At 24 years old, I was determined to learn the ropes of the natural health industry. My interests peaked where product formulation and branding was concerned. Being enrolled in the naturopathic doctor program, professors worked us to the bone mentally. Their curriculum included both western as well more traditional, eastern medical points of views. It's incredible how encompassing Traditional Chinese Medicine (TCM) is for example, considering both yin and yang components for achieving balance. Properties such as Cold and hot, slow and fast, solid versus fluid and energetic, were all considered, respectively. This way of thinking applies to all facets of TCM, from acupuncture to breathing, to herbal medicines. Angelica sinensis might be combined with Vastex agnis castis in a women's health formula, for instance. Cooling properties of liquorice might balance appropriately with warming effects of ginger and turmeric in the right amounts, and so forth.

Although many herbal extractions exist, with the natural health industry being confusing for many, I believe it's important to determine which core philosophy best embodies who you are, and what your goals entail. I'd like to spend a little bit of time sharing with you how I evaluate which herbal formulas are of top quality. First, it's important to understand that virtually any herb you choose, will unquestionably contain hundreds if not thousands of unique chemical/health promoting compounds, within. What those compounds do, are another story altogether. Needless to say, some mix well with water and others more so in fat, therefore each requiring different methods of extraction. You might be familiar with dark, liquid tinctures where herbs are immersed in a specific percentage of ethyl alcohol for a period of time. Although I never thought of tea or coffee as extractions, they most certainly are; hot water, chemical free, to be exact. Espresso incorporates both hot water as well as pressure, over time. Just a slight variation in any one variable will completely change the aroma, taste, and overall experience.

Most herbal formulas today, that you will find at the local health store for joints, hormones, liver, etc., involve what are referred to as 'standardized extractions'. These are a dime a dozen and almost always require harsh, chemical solvents. To give you an idea, acetone is nail polish remover and hexane, dry cleaning fluid. Yet, these are some of the most commonly used. Oh, and by the way, it doesn't stop at herbal formulas. Your greens supplements that you think of as being so incredibly healthy, more often than not will have these types of extracts within or involve chemical gas sprays, converting the fruits and vegetables into a dried powder form. Although innovative companies are implementing chemical free methods of accomplishing the same or better results, they are few and far between. Supercritical uses carbon dioxide with pressure, over time, requiring a tremendous amount of expertise. Freeze drying methods is another great distinction worth voting with your dollar for. While, these chemical free methods yield a full spectrum of healing compounds, standardization does not. This is where your philosophy matters.

What you believe, matters. Will your body receive the most benefit from the infinite wisdom of all compounds contained within a herb, or from one unique molecule, which has been ripped out, acting more as a drug? Standardized extracts are the latter in my opinion, indeed evidenced based, capitalizing on what some believe to be active compounds within a given herb, however controversial to say the least. L-theanine and ECGC are two unique examples, which are ripped out of green tea and sold everywhere. Although having great potential as far as research is concerned thus far, there are a multitude of other compounds in the same herb, waiting their turn to be discovered. Furthermore, inherent synergy exists in how various compounds interact with each other, not just in terms of efficacy, but in terms of safety as well, wouldn't you agree? Full spectrum, chemical free extractions combine science with ancient wisdom. Nevertheless, the choice is up to you.

Working in a small, 600 square foot, local health food store, was somewhat of an apprenticeship. I learned that not all companies are created equally as some are innovative, while most fall short as copycats. One of my mentors and I refer to these as "me too" brands. With a passion for learning, hundreds of brands and maybe thousands of formulas were candy for my curiosity craving. I've learned that one person's idea of quality, might not resonate with someone else's. Some formulas were well thought out and others had major flaws. Some were current in consumer buying trends, and there were even those which I suspect created some of the buying trends in the first place. As my imagination often went wild, I even envisioned what my own product formulas would entail.

Nothing peaked my interest more, however than sports supplements. The marketing got to me, no question. Packaging materials and colours were and still are incredibly eye catching. Textures are cutting edge, designed with specific consumers in mind. Competitive bodybuilders typically in their peak condition right after a contest, are integrated into label designs. The shier language, pertaining to extreme results that no one ever sees simply by taking supplements on their own, are well thought out. Everything about these products are created to gear up the senses and make you, the consumer, a believer; if you buy their product, you can be a bodybuilder too.

Many products on a shelf are not Health Canada compliant. Should that surprise you? After all, a messy restroom tells you something about the kitchen, right? Many labels don't even have the courtesy of listing both official languages of Canada; how dare they. Imagine how confusing the shopping experience is for American shoppers, where competition is even fiercer. Third party tests, balanced ingredients, and quality of ingredients are absent in an overwhelming number of products within the industry, yet even more so within the sports nutrition category. Artificial flavours and colourings are only part of the problem.

It's no secret that the natural health industry has its fair share of skeptics, often criticizing the lack of scientific research, so what is one to think when looking at a sports supplement? You need not go further than most pre-workout formulas, which contain dangerously high amounts of stimulants, which are accompanied by a long list of isolated, compounds, with sketchy science that no one has ever heard of. That said, some companies are fantastic examples by which others should model their approach by. Consumers simply need to become more savvy if quality and efficacy are important proponents of what they are looking for. GMP (Good Manufacturing Process) certification is a distinction worth considering and if you're looking for more premium designations, certified organic and Non-GMO Project verified, will say a lot about a brand's commitment to quality.

By far, some of the top selling products where I worked, were protein powders. These days, you will often see entire walls of a store dedicated to huge tubs worth. As with herbs, different versions of quality persist in the marketplace and it's important to decide which version is right for you. In the case of protein powder labels, you'll inevitably be faced with the question of what product is of higher quality; whey protein concentrate or isolate? If the majority of your shopping experience is within mass market, at least up until maybe the last 3 years or so ago, most of the protein powders that you've been exposed to were either labeled as "whey protein concentrate," or some of the perceived higher quality products were a blend of both, often with the addition of egg, dairy, soy, and pea protein.

Whey is a product of the dairy industry, and marketed as a fantastic way for people to bridge the gap of what might be missing in their diet. After all, the body uses protein for pretty much everything as a basic building block, doesn't it? Powders have and absolutely will never replace the nutritional value of genuine, whole food, whether plant or animal based. There is absolutely no comparison for many reasons, however companies spend lots of time and money trying to create false needs convincing people otherwise. Many of us are now familiar with absorption, for instance. With digestive concerns affecting so many, not everyone is absorbing as much nutrition from their diet as they should. Therefore, they should be filling that gap with nutritional supplements, instead of addressing the root cause of malabsorption in the first place. This is of course non-sense. Many protein powder companies take a similar approach and use food comparisons right on their marketing material. You are likely to absorb higher amounts of protein from whey isolate than a generous piece of steak, chicken, or pork and so buying their product provides a fantastic solution;

or does it? Should we choose powder over food? No. Absorption isn't everything.

Whey concentrate absorbs at a slower rate than isolates and contain relatively high amounts of cholesterol. I was both impressed and shocked while reading 55mg on some labels, realizing that many people unknowingly consume double and triple the recommended serving size. I mean; why wouldn't they, right? In a wholesome shake, adding extra scoops of powder is not only easy, but adds tremendous flavour. Although there is more cholesterol in one egg yolk, it all adds up. Being mindful of label ingredients and amounts is surely worthwhile.

Whey protein isolates are even more highly processed, which means arguably more chemical interventions. However, the end result in this case, is an amino acid product whereby the absorption is much higher and cholesterol content is zero or negligible. Plus, the relatively low calorie and carbohydrate content, serves as a potential strategy in overcoming cravings, thus achieving longer, sustained energy. In some cases, you may choose one over the other merely according to what fitness goals you're trying to achieve.

We sold mostly whey protein isolates at the store where I worked, yet I have had the pleasure of hearing arguments on both sides. The 'concentrate' people value their slower absorption and insist, "if you want to gain muscle while you sleep, which is when we are truly repairing at our pinnacle, then having a slower, sustained released will help keep the body in an anabolic (building [muscle]) state." The 'isolate' people countered with "are you kidding? That's them trying to sell you the cheap stuff. Protein isolate requires more processing, is more expensive, and they are simply trying to sell against the fact that they are using outdated technology." Then they'd really get savvy and elaborate, "besides, if you really want sustained release, then you can just mix our whey isolate in a glass of milk before bed and ba-baam, you'd have your sustained release without compromising quality and innovation." This was pretty much the exact conversation that I had with two sales reps of different companies, with the exception that neither of them said "ba-baam".

Without picking apart every protein supplement on the market, I was intrigued to divert my attention to mass gainers. At first the idea was peculiar. Mass gainer? Isn't the goal of most of us to actually lose weight? Why would anyone want to pay good money for this nonsense? First of all, someone with cachexia, where the body might be wasting from diseases such as cancer or AIDS, may benefit in some way from consuming as many calories as possible, especially when appetite and general consumption rate is at an all-time low.[1,2] Second, mass gainers are marketed towards building bulk muscle mass. Most top level professional bodybuilders are generous enough to share the single best way to accomplish that; through eating high amounts of real, whole food. The late Rich Piana of 5% Nutrition, is one such bodybuilder who fully acknowledges, after working for protein powder companies, although these items can certainly offer value in certain instances, the best approach is by far that which real food is the staple.[3] If significant muscle gains still are not reached, despite working out intensely and eating 6-8 meals per day, Rich will gladly advise increasing further, the time spent in the gym as well as food intake to as many as 10-12 meals per day. He has recommended this time and time again before ever resorting to a powder, which is starting to become the current trend among some of the most successful athletes.

Food might be perceived as expensive for many, and meal prep daunting when implemented on a consistent basis, but these are all excuses. More so for convenience, as well as appetite and digestive issues, I agree that mass gainer supplements may certainly have their place. While evaluating probably the single most successful weight gainer brand that I've seen, I noticed something on the label that took my breath away. Saturated fat content in a natural health product! I was shocked and concerned. How could this be? I contacted the company to inquire further and was inspired; coconut oil's medium chain triglycerides (MCT) have a greater propensity towards energy usage, rather than as a way of shortening the path towards cholesterol heaven. The MCT revolution began to finally make sense. It was all about energy.

Medium Chain Triglycerides are marketed as being an active ingredient from coconut oil, leading people into believing that isolated MCT products are therefore super concentrated, potent versions of whole, raw coconut oil. While the whole food has nutritional value, people are sold on false promises that MCT isolates are more therapeutic. Do you see a pattern emerging within the industry? Isolates versus the whole; which one is better? Ultimately that's for you to decide, however I will say this; an MCT product is no coconut oil.

MCT isolates are highly processed, using chemicals and lack vitality, the very essence of its claim. Coconut oil conversely, has antimicrobial properties, interestingly enough against fungus, notably Candida albicans. The whole, raw oil is rich in various nutrients and compounds, which contribute to areas of immune health, providing antioxidants, all while tasting fantastic. Moderation however is still key, as if the recent Coca Cola television commercial on weight gain has taught me anything, it is that "all calories count, no matter where they come from."[4]

Just because something in moderation is great for you, doesn't mean that in excess this still holds true. As in the case of my Mom warning me against eating too much Chinese Food, Sushi, and Thai, even the latter which is often viewed by many health advocates as the healthier choice, I'm urging you not to be fooled as they have been. After all, what would their spicy chicken dish taste like without an abundance of sodium? If Pad Thai weren't loaded with sugar, would you order it? Let's not forget about MSG loaded fish sauce. With a love for

Thai coconut curries, I insist the saturated fat (MCTs) contained within, isn't as bad for my cholesterol as Mom previously thought. Nevertheless, she cautions portion size, and I agree.

Using a measuring spoon and cup will certainly clear up any doubts as to whether coconut curry fits in with your daily caloric goals. If you are reducing other oils to make room for this one, while maintaining a healthy weight, coconut oil can be an amazing option, which has a wide array of health promoting benefits. The real question, is whether you will switch from butter to solid, spreadable, coconut oil on your toast in the morning. No? I don't blame you. After all, they say butter makes it better, don't they? Then again, perhaps you're more of a margarine type.

Chapter 16:

Butter Makes It Better

Butter and passion go hand in hand. I suppose that when it comes down to it, the foods that I associate with containing the most butter, come from my grandmother's cooking. My kids are unbelievably lucky that they live in the same city as both sets of grandparents. My brothers and I on the other hand, didn't have that luxury. Growing up, my Dad's parents lived in Montreal and my Mom's in Winnipeg, so we were lucky if we saw them every 4-6 months. When we were finally together, time flew, yet each and every time became harder to say goodbye, especially as they got older and we started to become more cognizant of the fact that at some point, it may be our last.

There is an emotional link to food, no question. There are those foods, which just always seem to taste better when prepared by someone special, aren't there? One of my favourite all-time foods is cabbage rolls and to be honest I don't even think my grandmother actually included butter whatsoever. That said, when I think of butter, the first thought that pops in my head is the buttery goodness of those one of a kind cabbage rolls. I've ordered them in countless places, yet most use larger amounts of rice as filler. Bubby's rolls were mostly meat, tender as can be, with a thin, but not too thin, red tomato sauce, which was a little peppery but ultimately sweet and slightly tangy. My Dad admits she probably added sugar.

I used to call them up every week like clockwork, and to this day I regret the one time I asked Bubby to make extra cabbage rolls, which I loved so much. Driving 6 hours from Montreal to Toronto, her and Zaidy used to drive with their car jam packed with Tupperware® containers full of food. This one particular visit, she must have made enough to tie us over until their next trip. I ate so many that I actually became sick of them; something that I can't even fathom at the moment, though I unfortunately told her, nevertheless. My knees are becoming weak just at these words pouring out over this page. Cabbage rolls are not easy to make by the way. They require an abundance of time and even though there are certain tricks, making peeling off layers easier, such as pre-boiling, make no mistake they're a lot of work. Not that Bubby minded. After all, our ear to ear smiles after our first bite in 4 months, were priceless.

My intention was to give her a break, as it pained me knowing that she was getting older and cooking was becoming increasingly difficult. I wish to this day that I would have just shut my mouth, because not a day goes by, where I don't think of her and those mind boggling good, one of a kind, buttery cabbage rolls. It's the difference between real and authentic, and all of the other noise out there. That pretty much unto itself, sums up how I feel about the difference between butter and margarine. Emotional and authentic, versus whatever it is that you think margarine is.

I suppose that when we have an emotional connection with food and the way that we eat it, the thought of not over indulging, can be difficult to say the least. I believe that's what happened with the butter versus margarine dilemma. Butter has a taste unlike anything else, doesn't it? It makes great sauces and I'm not just talking about creamy Alfredo or as part of a wine reduction. In fact, I recently learned that it's one of the main ingredients to caramel sauce; who knew? From cakes to cookies, to beautiful, delicate croissants, butter is an essential and amazing ingredient, in many deserts. Then again, how about a dollop over top of steamed veggies? What's a baked potato without butter and chives? Brussel's Sprouts were always a favourite of mine growing up, without any seasoning. Little did I know, that adding a little bit of butter over top would send my taste buds on a voyage to another dimension of flavour.

I made a huge mistake, fresh out of school, while at a best friend's house for dinner. His father had high cholesterol and I'm not sure why we happened to be speaking about it at the dinner table, but he shared with me that he had been taking Lipitor® to control it. Me in my over confidence, shared with him that I now had the knowledge, that could possibly get him off his medication while still controlling and maintaining healthy cholesterol levels, but that I knew, in my arrogance, that he wouldn't go for it. His father is a very smart, proud man, with great taste in food, music, and cars. The care that he puts into his car and his stereo system is a sight, let me tell you. In the summers of the late 90's, my friend and I would walk back to his place from the local mall only to see his father, not cleaning, but caressing his Black, Pontiac TransAm. He exercised regularly and was by no means over weight; in fact, he was and still is, in fantastic shape. Still, his high cholesterol was something that surely I thought he could take more seriously and I was the man for the job. This was my opportunity to give back for all his family's hospitality over the years.

My friend's father said "Come on Rob, just tell me. It can't be that bad". I replied in an intentional but nevertheless snobby tone with "you wouldn't go through it anyway. It's just too hard, so why don't you let me know when you're really serious about lowering your cholesterol and we can meet up and I'll tell you everything." He looked at me, seeing right through my act and said "Just tell me, seriously I want to know". So I let him in on a few foods, amounts, and supplements that he'd need to take, followed by the 'unfortunate news' that he needed to really cut out as much cholesterol as possible. By the way, for the record, we don't even need cholesterol from our food, as if you recall, most of the cholesterol that we use is actually produced by our liver. We're fine without it, but man oh man, it is heavenly; I know.

We spoke briefly about several food items such certain dairy products as well as amounts of cholesterol that he should be cognizant of on food labels, which I'll be diving into shortly. Chicken wings, and certain cuts of steak were difficult but doable, but wow when I arrived at butter, let me tell you; it was like taking the shirt right off the gentleman's back. It was as if I broke one of his wings and he lost his ability to fly. "Are you crazy?" he said. Actually in all reality it's been so long now that I'm not sure that's exactly what he said but I'm hearing his voice in my head right now.

Suddenly, my friend's mother begins bringing dinner to the table. They're an Armenian family with the majority of their cooking having a large Iranian influence, passed down from my friend's grandmother to his mother. The spices and care that go into their food reminds me of my grandparents even though they're from completely different cultures. I know it sounds emotional, because I'm an emotional kind of a guy, but the love that goes into that type of food is something out of this world. Rice is presented on a massive bowl, family style, in the middle of the table. The individual plates that they have aren't round like 'normal' plates that I have at my home, but rather oval so that you can pile on a massive amount of beautifully, scented, long grain, basmati rice before then placing the meat over top.

The rice has a hint of yellow which is either from turmeric or saffron, or a combination of the two. You know when food is perfectly seasoned when you're salivating on the thought of your second helping, yet not even finished the first bite. Once lightly salted, a generous portion of butter is placed over top, melting every so softly due to the piping hot steam. As we're talking, we all kind of pause and stare at the rice in awe. As my friend's father offered us first dibs, we all fill our places and then just pause again. I looked right up at him after just taking in the aromas, we pause, he looked back down at the rice, places some in his spoon and before eating, looks right at me and exclaims "you want me, to give up, this?!" That's when it really hit how foolish and naive I was. There's of course a much better way of maintaining healthy cholesterol than to simply cut all of it out. Still, in a society where we simply eat too much of it, people wanted a healthy alternative that looked and tasted sort of like butter, but whether we succeeded, is another question.

We as a society are so incredibly obsessed with butter as being a solid, spreadable oil, that just the thought of having to give it up for the sake of the high cholesterol epidemic, drove us out of our minds, to the point that we literally had to invent a synthetic, butter alternative, called margarine. Can you imagine? This was an absolutely ingenious idea, all thanks to a process called hydrogenation. Saturated fat like butter and lard are solid at room temperatures, but unsaturated fats like vegetable oils are liquid. It was discovered that if you chemically alter vegetable oils to add hydrogen molecules to their structures, through freakish scientific experimentation, you could literally convert liquid vegetable oils into solid, spreadable awesomeness. Margarine was born. Sounds amazing, doesn't it? There were a few things wrong with it, however.

When looking at the chemical structure of margarine, it turns out that the arrangement of the hydrogen atoms matter, big time. During the process of hydrogenation, some of the hydrogen atoms flip one way, and others another. Depending on how they're flipped, they're called either trans or cis formations. Scientific research has demonstrated repeatedly that trans-fat intake, such as the ones produced within margarine, dramatically increase cardiovascular disease risk and we are only beginning to understand why. We know that it has the ability to increase LDL cholesterol and lower HDL cholesterol, much like saturated fat. It can be found in fried foods so watch out for donuts, fries, and partially hydrogenated vegetable oils.[1]

What's important to know, is that packaged goods such as some cookies and other baked items, contain some trans fats so reading labels are important. Simply look for zero trans fats on the label and avoid it like the plague. Without going into too much detail, this problem was addressed and solved. Even writing that, I'm absolutely amazed at our resourcefulness, aren't you? I mean we were absolutely determined to find a 'healthy' butter alternative so that we could have our spread on toast without the risk of cardiovascular disease.

Companies developed non-hydrogenated margarines, which are what you'll mostly find these days in grocery stores. They are trans-fat free or dramatically low in trans-fat. The New York City Health Code, Section 81.08 states that there is no harmless level of artificial trans-fat consumption, whatsoever. There are also no, known health benefits, which is why this is one fat, which should truly and completely be eliminated from our diets. So what exactly is the problem with margarines today, you might ask? It comes down to processing and ingredients once again. If you scroll down the ingredient list, you'll notice that while butter really only has cream (more on this later) and maybe milk in the ingredient list, margarine on the other hand has many more, not to mention, there is an underlying point, which I'll dive into now.

Here are the ingredients of a typical margarine:

1. Canola and sunflower oils 74%
2. Water
3. Modified palm and palm kernel oils 6%
4. Salt 1.8%
5. Whey protein concentrate 1.4%
6. Soy lecithin 0.2%
7. Vegetable monoglycerides
8. Potassium sorbate
9. Vegetable colour
10. Artificial flavor
11. Citric acid
12. Vitamin A palmitate
13. Vitamin D3
14. Alpha-tocopherol acetate (vitamin E)

Note: I have purposely left out the source of this ingredient list in fairness to the specific brand that I selected randomly from my grocery shelf.

I encourage you to simply head over to the store and choose any non-hydrogenated margarine that you'd like and compare. They don't have to be exactly the same. In fact, I'm not even going to spend too much time picking apart the controversies of every single ingredient, as I feel as though most of them are either truly insignificant or even if that seems like an outrage to you, they still sort of miss the real point. I'll explain further.

It truly comes down to fortified vitamins, artificial flavour, highly processed, isolates, and possibly genetically modified ingredients, which aren't specifically labeled as such. In fact, it's not even fair to attack margarine for these, as many processed, packaged food items contain them. Citric acid is typically used as a preservative, while artificial flavour is truly a category in its own right. In fact, I honestly have no idea what it can possibly mean, although any of us can simply look it up on google and obtain a wide array of possibilities. Better to avoid it altogether, don't you think? Vegetable monoglycerides are typically isolated from corn, and probably genetically modified, though we'd never know it due to labelling not being mandatory here in North America. This is where Europe is far ahead of us in terms of consumer food transparency. [2] Potassium sorbate, although is used against oxidation for the purpose of preserving flavour, colour, and preventing mould growth, not a whole lot is known. One Turkish study in 2009 suggest genotoxicity in human blood lymphocytes in vitro (so not actually tested in humans)[3], yet a more comprehensive review can be found at this footnote here.[4] Vegetable colour can be any number of things as it does not explicitly say.

Now that we've gone through the list, we can focus on the only ingredients that actually have any real percentage stake. We assume these are the ingredients, which are in higher, relative amounts. This of course doesn't necessarily mean much, as a very tiny amount of a really bad chemical, can still do a lot of harm. Still, if you've ever consumed a whey protein powder, chances are, you've consumed quite a bit of whey protein concentrate, not to mention that it's an ingredient used in many consumer food items, so I'm not too worried about 1.4% of it. Soy lecithin comprises a small percentage, however soy in of itself isn't even necessarily that healthy for us. Soy is incredibly difficult to digest, contains a multitude of allergens, and that's really just part of the story.

The majority of soy here in North America is loaded with pesticides and is typically genetically modified, so if your intention is to avoid genetically modified foods, then soy is one to really pay attention to. It's interesting that herbicide amount actually increases in genetically modified corn and soy, as they have been altered specifically to handle more of it. [5] Furthermore, soy lecithin is an isolated substance, which means that in order to rip the lecithin from whole soy, a massive amount of processing needs to be performed, usually involving chemical solvents such as hexane, acetone, and bleaching compounds, to name a few. A 2013 study examined the effect of soy lecithin on depression, using albino rats. The conclusion is priceless: "Soy lecithin was successfully isolated economically from soy sludge and all parameters for which it was evaluated were within specified limits, except for benzene-insoluble compounds".[6] Great; benzene-insoluble compounds and sludge. Yummy. As Nick Stewart said in It's a Mad, Mad, Mad, Mad World; "I've said it before, and I'll say it again,"[7] there truly is no telling what these isolates will do in our bodies long term. Interestingly, soy lecithin is used in the supplement industry as a promoter of good overall health of the nervous system, including contributing to a nerve's myelin sheath. This is a focus on diseases such as Multiple Sclerosis. Either way, the amount contained in margarine is truly negligible.

The take home for modified palm and kernel oil, is exactly that; they're modified. You may read about the controversies pertaining to their saturated fat content, but with only 6% in this margarine, is it really anything worthwhile talking about? I think not. I mean, if you just use a dollop of cream in your coffee in the morning, then you shouldn't even bother looking at this ingredient here as it's a drop in the ocean. Finally, we arrive at the main ingredient which is nothing more than canola and sunflower oil. Here is where I hope to offer some true insight.

Both canola and sunflower oils are omega-6 essential fatty acids. You might remember that we as a society already probably consume way too much omega-6 but still, I have faith in you. I have faith that you're already beginning to dramatically reduce poor cooking methods of omega-6 and truly any fat for that matter, such as frying. The same holds true for packaged products high in vegetable oils, which may undergo processing involving high heat. In that case, adding small amounts of pure, uncooked omega-6 to your diet will probably only add value. Consuming way too much omega-6 relative to omega-3 (fish, chia, flax), is where an overabundance of inflammation can be ignited, which we want to try and avoid as much as possible.

In the case of margarine, these oils may be heated, though I will admit that canola and sunflower oils have a much higher smoke point than say olive oil. I realize there are other choices such as grape seed oil, avocado oil, and even coconut oil. Still, heating might not be the only process as harsh chemical solvents may be used as well. These are questions that I'd ask before purchasing a margarine if any of that concerns you. Here's my ultimate bottom line.

Knowing that canola and sunflower oils contribute to 74% of the product, which is definitely something to sneeze about, can't we just save ourselves the headache all together if we just settle on not having to purchase a solid, spreadable oil product in the first place? I mean, do you really need to be able to have a solid lump of oil? Can't you just purchase certified organic, Non-GMO Project Verified, sunflower or canola oil and call it a day? I think yes. In fact, that's exactly what I would do. If you want to avoid margarine but have the best of what margarine offers (which is not a whole lot by the way), why not grab a measuring spoon and drizzle some of the good stuff over your toast, rice, or salad? As a plus, oils taste much better raw as well.

The rare time that you actually do want to spread or add a little bit of butter to your food (and I'll repeat, "a little"), just do it. 1 tablespoon of butter is about 120kcal (1 tsp = 40kcal), just as any other oil. If your cholesterol is high, and 200mg is considered a high amount for someone trying to reduce their risk of cardiovascular disease, you have a nice base by which to go by. Adding 1tsp of butter once a week or so is less than moderate in my book, but again it's completely up for debate. The bottom line, is to truly place it in context with what you're eating. In the case of my friend's father, the butter wasn't the problem. I was naive in thinking he had to go to that extreme by completely eliminating it out of his diet to lower his cholesterol.

What he really needed to do, was take into account the possible chicken wings after work, the fatty salami on that snack platter at the office event, and the splashes of cream in 2-3 coffees per day. Let's not forget about the cheese that absolutely had to be in that fabulous triple decker, club sandwich. Finally, consider whether the 'small' slab of butter over rice is truly 'once in a while'. It doesn't look so glamorous for cholesterol now, does it? It's not our fault, as our grandparents knew more about this stuff than we did.

Our grandparents used pure, natural, real, whole food. They probably just used too much of certain ingredients, likely cooking them in unhealthy manners. This is the very reason why committing to your diet diary and seeking professional guidance is so valuable. If 'moderation' is something that you're unsure of, your diet diary will certainly shed some light, as you may be consuming cholesterol rich foods in much higher quantities that you realize. At the end of the day, consuming nutrient dense, real WHOLE foods that are mindful and helpful towards INFLAMMATION, STRESS, and ENERGY metabolism (WISE™ foods), not only help to keep cholesterol within healthy lab ranges but more importantly act to support the overall health of molecule itself. Remember, cholesterol is supposed to be on our side; we just need to take better care of it so that it functions properly.

Chapter 17:

Organic versus 'Conventional' Non-Organic

Our grandparents didn't really have organic, or rather organic was simply 'normal food'. Imagine going back in time and letting your grandparents or perhaps even their parents know that in the future, our farmers will purchase copious amounts of toxic chemical compounds and spray their crops to help keep bugs away. What do you think they would say? Perhaps that we're off our rocker? I think, maybe yes. Even now, living in this 'toxic world' of ours, when describing to someone what a genetically modified organism is for the first time, their expression is priceless.

"You're kidding," is pretty much the just of it. "You're telling me, that we as a society are buying corn, which contains genes of a toxin producing bacteria?" They ask. "Yup," I reply. They pause, and then continue with "Then this genetically modified corn has the ability to produce its own toxin, the same toxin that the bacteria produced, that can cause insects stomachs to explode?" "Yup", I reply again. Imagine when they learn about some of the sketchy science. We were told that they were proven to be safe, only to realize as early as 2012, when we eat GMO corn, the toxins are able to cause inflammation in our digestive tracts, notably our microvilli, which help with absorption of nutrients. There have been major correlations between increased autoimmune conditions and food sensitivities since the introduction of GMOs into the marketplace.[1]

There is a fantastic documentary called *Genetic Roulette: The Gamble of Our Lives* by Jeffrey M. Smith, which explains this all in much more detail. Whether you are for or against GMOs is not really the issue in a way, but would you agree that at least they should be listed on food labels? Our grand or great grandparents would surely warn us; food should be grown without the use of chemicals from the ground, the way nature intended. Now, I am not a purist by any means, despite my efforts to live as healthy of a lifestyle as possible within what I perceive as moderation. I have my moments and you may very well find me running in to pick up take out somewhere. It's possible, I'm not going to lie; don't judge me.

I realize full well that in certain parts of the world, famine, weather patterns, and soil quality are major issues, along with political instability, which don't afford the same luxuries as we do with respect to farming practices. There are valid arguments on both sides. Still, here's the perceived scam as far as organic is concerned. Paying six dollars for 12 organic eggs when we can pay half that for non-organic. Nine dollars for 2L of organic milk versus half that for regular. Berries are an absolute joke, aren't they? Three dollars for one measly cucumber appears hardly fair, simply because it says organic on it. We all have mouths to feed and I completely understand.

If produce is considered pricey, meat will surely be perceived as breaking the bank. Twenty dollars for one, smaller sized chicken is one great example. Many are convinced that organic is just a marketing scam as how can certification agencies be trusted? Lastly, as far as global farming is concerned, many are not convinced that organic practices provide sufficient crop yields. Now, let's discuss why considering organic is more than worthwhile.

It's certainly important not to be naive as some items are plain rip-offs. Gauging; I'm the first one to admit. That said, there are still many worthy of switching over to organic. Sure there are lists of 'top dirty dozen' plastered all over the web, but here is the cream of the crop. Seriously; have you ever read the ingredient list on your cream? Everyone knows how much I love coffee; the daily grind as you may call it. As I mentioned, I never used cream prior to meeting my wife, merely due to the high fat content, though honestly we all know how unbelievable it tastes. Having always been a 2% man, I woke up one morning about 6-8 months ago contemplating that fat aside, maybe the actual concept of using cream is in some way healthier, at least from a synergy point of view. After all, cream is more whole than some fractionated percentage of milk, isn't it? This thought process let me to the notion that just maybe there would be some health benefits, which I could gain in extreme moderation. At least this was how I legitimized my taste buds' dream.

While feeling so proud of myself for this incredible epiphany, I went out and bought 10% half and half cream. When I got home, I read the ingredients. Here they are and again no reference necessary as I dare you to just walk over to your fridge or the nearest store and check it out for yourself, regardless of most brands.

10% Half and Half:

1. Milk

2. Cream

3. Sodium Citrate

4. Sodium Phosphate

5. Carrageenan

Table Cream:

1. Milk
2. Cream
3. Sodium Citrate
4. Sodium Phosphate
5. Carrageenan

Whipping Cream:

1. Cream
2. Milk
3. Carrageenan
4. Mono and Dyglycerides
5. Carboxymethyl Cellulose
6. Polysorbate 80

I couldn't believe my eyes. Can you? It was at this point that I frantically looked for the organic version to see if there was a difference at least as far as the label was concerned. Finally, I found 10% half and half organic cream. Guess what the ingredients are?

Organic 10% Half and Half:

1. Milk
2. Cream

I know that the price is pretty much double and we shouldn't have to pay that. Organic shouldn't be special; it should be what 'normal' food is called. However, the truth is that it's not. We live in a world where the simple ingredients our grandmothers used, now come from highly processed, isolated chemicals, which are from highly manipulated, genetically modified foods such as corn. Mono and diglycerides, and maltodextrin are merely two such examples. Have you looked at the tub of frozen yogurt or ice cream in your freezer? Have a look, g'ahead. I dare you. Sure organic is double the price, but at the end of the day, have you ever considered that it's still just a matter of a few dollars? Do you not deserve dairy, free of these additional chemicals for $5.00 extra?

Whether 25 cents or 50 cents per egg, at the end of the day, six dollars for an organic dozen is really just about a dollar for a 2 egg breakfast. Sure it's double, but do you not deserve to spend a buck for eggs that have been laid by chickens who were free to roam around, fed good quality foods themselves, and were free from hormone and antibiotics? With respect to chemically sprayed produce, even if organic kale is five dollars compared to its 'conventional', for three bucks, shouldn't you and your family enjoy fewer chemicals if reasonable? Even if someone proved to you that indeed there are chemical residues despite what the certification agencies claim. If they showed you that it was dramatically less than the regular stuff, would you not buy it? Just offering some perspective.

Whole fat forms of dairy in high amounts over time, such as cream and butter, rich in saturated fat, can negatively impact cholesterol as well as triglyceride levels. Therefore, I'm in no way advocating their consumption. However, they are phenomenal energy sources and mounting evidence suggests that the type of feed matters within an animal's diet and their respective milk supply attributes; not to mention the quality of life for the animal. Some research suggests that a diet rich in grass can favourably alter an animal's fatty acid balance towards an ideal omega-6 to omega-3 ratio, as well as increase the amount of beta-carotene, vitamin A and vitamin E within a cow's milk supply, naturally. Don't you find it odd, that some of these are actually added to 'normal' milk?[2,3] Although these variables may not affect the quantity of cholesterol and triglycerides contained within, it might have more favourable impacts as far as other risk factors for cardiovascular disease go, such as inflammation. The difference between Grass Fed and Organic, just in case you are wondering, is that the cow's continually roam freely as they feed in the first, whereas not necessarily year round in the latter.

My bottom line, is that butter and cream, if consumed, moderation needs to be exercised and the same holds true for any cholesterol containing food. Avoiding as much as possible, the oxidizing of the product, visa vie cooking on high heat or high enough to cause browning/smoking. Moreover, metabolic oxidative stress needs to be taken into consideration (oxidation within the body, naturally due to stress of all kinds; immune, emotional, physical, etc.). Furthermore, organic may be a better option than the regular conventional varieties. Personally, I'd love more third party chemical analysis, resulting in more information present on food labels. However, there is still a lot to be gained from common sense, label reading. By the way, not everything I eat is organic or local. I pick and choose just like the next person, but as we become more informed, each of us can begin to make our own decisions regarding our nutrition and place value on what matters most to each of us.

How to Find Time to Eat Healthy

One of the greatest challenges standing in the way of eating healthy, is time. A purist might argue "well that's just laziness". Luckily, I'm here to settle this once and for all; it is not laziness. The opposite is true, as people are over-worked, if anything. Several years ago, my brother-in-law enthused me into watching a diet and exercise video series, promising results in the way of a ripped physique. Preparing many meals in advance, was the take home, and although neglected by many, amongst bodybuilders, this is both common knowledge and practice. After all; eating large volumes of calculated food per day is mandatory for gaining muscle mass. Surprisingly, their meal size is often smaller than what an average person might imagine, as too much food in one sitting results in bloating and indigestion, which is counterproductive in achieving an athletic looking tiny waist with massive, muscular limbs, known as the 'x-frame'.

Whereas an average person may eat about 3 large meals per day with some snacks in between, bodybuilders eat as much as 5-7 for maintenance and up to 10-12 small to medium size meals when bulking up for a trade-show or contest. Meal preparation becomes daunting but dedication conquers all. Incredible merit lies in our ability to scale this idea to our own standard of living. As we proceed towards my grocery store walk through, the notion of advanced meal preparation needs to be front of mind, with 3-4 days' worth of prepping as the absolute minimum. This ensures your meals are well calculated, keeping your nutrition goals on track, while freeing up time.

Simple recipes are time consuming at home, yet ready in no time by a trained chef. In addition to experience, I presume the disconnect likely resides in preparation. Storing pre-cut ingredients ahead of time in glass containers such as Pyrex® is a great way to bridge that gap. The only challenge standing between you and your next fresh, crisp salad, is choosing which savoury, pre-made mason jar dressing you should drizzle over top, using a measuring spoon. A pair of scissors seamlessly cuts entire packages of oven baked chicken breasts into small cubes for later use. Inexpensive rice cookers provide 40 fragrant half-cup portions, while perfectly taking out the guess work. Leftovers will never taste the same as on the first day you prepare something, however as a helpful reminder, days 2-5 taste identical. Moreover, there are instances such as with soups, stew, and chilies, where flavours actually further develop over longer periods of time.

I find it helpful to think about the time meal prepping ultimately frees up. After all, time is the most valuable asset we own, isn't it? Perhaps a trip to the gym or colouring with your kids makes it worthwhile. Catching up on your favourite television program is just one prep day away from becoming a reality. You've been meaning to indulge in your favourite hobby, yet unable to until now. Earlier nights for better quality rest is suddenly a dream come true. Think about it this way; planning meals during your sharpest hours, offers you at your best, for those times if and when you become tempted to slip. This system empowers you to create your own delicious, mouth-watering recipes based on your shopping lists, without ever having to rely on someone else's. Incorporating what you've learned from your personal diet diary, while choosing WISE™ foods, the power to promote lifelong wellness through knowledge that heals truly resides within you.

Chapter 18:

Grocery Walk Through

The grocery store is where most injuries happen. Would you buy into that as a somewhat fair statement? A Chiropractor once shared with me that the bread and butter of his practice was primarily shoulder and back injuries, which most often either originated from the gym down the street, or reoccurred there. This seemed peculiar to me, as intuitively, I assume that gyms are in fact places for rehabilitation, if anything. A place where for the most part, members really want to be, as it takes a certain mindset and time out of their day. A quote written on the wall of the gym where I work out say "If I could get only one message across to you, it would this: there are no right or wrongs about looking or feeling good." — David Patchell-Evans. No matter what level of success an athlete aspires to, there are always negative people that seem to find them, but hopefully never shake their confidence.

In following some professional athletes on social media, I often read comments full of positivity, support, and enthusiasm for respective accomplishments. That said, I don't think I will ever be desensitized to those, which are reserved for unnecessary criticism and belittlement. I admire people who genuinely intend to add value to others around them, aspiring to inspire. Learning from someone who is more advanced in any area than you, is uplifting. One of my professors started a class by admitting, with as many years under his belt, the more knowledge he accumulated, the notion that the less he really knew, become evidently clearer.

In a gym setting, experts and amateurs alike are often more than willing to lend a hand. Still, there are times when being helpful masks someone's true intention of elevating personal ego. An expert may say "It blows me away, how many people come in here and perform this exercise wrong." At times I personally have witnessed an insulting "If you're going to come in here, do it right or not at all." Fears of judgment only act as roadblocks to enhanced performance, leading to greater risk of injury. No one joins a gym with the intention of performing an exercise incorrectly. I acknowledge the same truth as far as conscious grocery shopping is concerned and commend anyone who is doing their best to shop as WISE™ as possible.

Injury at the grocery store is not referring to a shopping cart accident or slippage. Rather I'm illuminating the deleterious effects that food can have on our bodies if we are not careful. However, I realize the level of effort required to make informed decisions. We are all doing the best that we can, particularly when in-store marketing is designed to sell product. The bottom line for any amazing grocery store educational walk through is really to instill the idea of perimeter shopping. The best way to prevent 'injury' in my opinion is to stay as much as possible along the outer sections rather than the inside. To be more specific, to stay within the fresh produce section rather than the inside isles, typically containing items such as cookies, crackers, cake, candies, condiments.

In effect, a grocery store is almost like one big medicine cabinet full of various labels that can be difficult to understand without a certain level of expertise. I can't think of a better place to exemplify the famous Socrates quote of 'let medicine be they food and food be thy medicine' other than perhaps the kitchen, though make no mistake, take the wrong pill, at the wrong dose, in the wrong combination, and accidents will happen. If you are like me and prefer not to indulge in a particular food, then don't buy it in the first place. A house void of potato chips or soda is less opportunity to splurge. Easier said than done. You invite friends over for dinner who arrive with a nice gesture, desert. Don't be afraid to let your guests know that you are really placing your health as priority and are setting goals. Letting them know how much their support means, will empower and inspire them. Explain that you avoiding sugary, fatty, packaged foods, snacks, or deserts in the home, while making WISE™ food choices.

Having the wrong foods in the house may seem harmless, but add up. Here's how. Your friends bring over a small cheesecake. No big deal. You prepared a WISE™ meal, leaving your guests feeling modestly full, yet more than satisfied and energized. Still, not to be rude, two slices of cake are modestly shared, leaving most of the cake still intact. What are you going to do? You wouldn't dream of throwing it away, would you? Do you know how many starving children there are in the world? You decide to keep the cake, slowly nibbling away throughout the week, feeling as if everything is under control. Sound familiar? Preaching to the choir.

Daily cholesterol recommendations are between 200-300mg based on cardiovascular disease risk factors. I believe 1-2 eggs every few days can add tremendous nutritional value, if we are WISE™ about not over cooking the 186mg or so of cholesterol contained within the yolk. Over easy, sunny side up, or poached are my favourite methods. The risk of cholesterol becoming oxidized once inside the body is still very real. Pre-existing inflammation is one example. Adding an antioxidant rich herb such as oregano or dill not only adds flavour but is a WISE™ choice, as is choosing eggs that may promote a balanced essential fatty acid intake.

Omega-3 enriched eggs may help sway inflammation or more specifically, arachidonic acid production in favour of balance. It is paramount that we consider the quality and care of animal farming practices. In the same way that WISE™ foods can influence our immune/inflammation/stress response, antioxidant defenses, and energy metabolism, the same hold true for animals. An earlier example of grass fed cows portrays the difference between dairy supporting us one way versus another. Eggs are no different.

Oils that are fed to animals often go rancid. In the same way that rancidity negatively affect our immune and inflammatory pathways, so do they affect animals' and thus the final product.[1,2] Livestock that are kept in close quarters, have an increased propensity for illness, requiring proactive measures such as frequent antibiotic use. Certified organic and grass fed distinctions are worthwhile though expensive. As a reasonable alternative, purchasing meat that states "without antibiotic use" likely correlates to higher quality farming practices in my opinion.

While shopping for food, I'm cognizant of my daily egg intake on average of 1 per day. That leaves me with little room for other cholesterol containing foods. Even a lean meat choice such as chicken breast contains about 100mg, so I have already reached my cholesterol limit for the day prior to even walking into a store. As a general rule of thumb, I rarely purchase anything that has more than 5-10mg of cholesterol per serving. In my opinion, if you stay clear of fatty meats, cheeses, and ice creams, you will find that a low cholesterol intake is fairly easy. As far as other forms of dairy are concerned, Kefir contains about 25mg per cup, which is a large serving. Organic, 2% milk contains about 20mg per cup, and cottage cheese a mere 10mg while providing an impressive 15g of protein. Greek yogurt will often yield 18g-22g of protein per cup while contributing a mere 10mg of cholesterol.

The remainder of your shopping list should really comprise of nutrient dense, WISE™ foods. Since 80% or so of cholesterol is produced by our livers and not from our diet, supporting liver function is also paramount. I find it interesting that many natural substances which have been found to ameliorate elevated cholesterol, often have coexisting liver protective properties, such as certain species of asparagus[3], Moringa oleifera leaf extract[4],

turmeric and garlic[5], artichoke[6], milk thistle[7], among others. Not to worry if you don't consume these on a regular basis, because as it turns out, the same holds true for many WISE™ foods, some of which we will discuss now.

To Juice or to Blend?

Fruits and vegetables are almost always located near the entrance of a grocery store. This is where the bulk of your time should be spent. Although this may seem intuitive, I would like to place emphasis on fibre, which has been used to dramatically help lower elevated cholesterol levels. Although I prefer and have recommended between 20-30g per day to my patients, anywhere from 5-25g is substantiated in the literature. One of my favourite approaches to increasing daily fibre intake includes delicious blended "green" smoothies.

There are two types of fibre; soluble and insoluble, where both provide various health benefits. For cholesterol maintenance, soluble fibre is the champion's choice.[8] Still, insoluble helps with digestion and overall health of the gut. By adhering to a large variety of whole foods, notably vegetables, you will have very little reason to worry one way or another. Variety is key.

Juicing has also received much attention in recent years, often in fad weight loss diets and health crazes for valid reasons. Both juicing and blending are incredible ways of obtaining high levels of nutrition in one beverage. Spending $400 on a juicer or $500 on a blender can be intimidating for many, to say the least. High quality juicers yield higher amount of nutrients from fruits and vegetables per glass than pretty much any other method, including blending. Extracting juice, while leaving behind pulp results in higher levels antioxidants, vitamins and minerals and other unique healing compounds.

Juice is only as good as the ingredients that are used. Therefore, simply adding large amounts of sweet, delicious fruit, reminds me of someone eating a Snicker's bar, saying "I'm receiving protein from the peanuts". Adding nutrient dense, liver protective, green, leafy vegetables, is absolutely the way to go in my opinion. However not all machines are capable of such a feat, as advanced grinding mechanisms are often required. This rationales the steep price point of entry level, high quality juicers such as the Omega VRT 350.

Despite thoroughly enjoying drinking fresh, green juices, my machine does not receive much attention these days. Simply put, I prefer not to throw away the pulp. Experts will explain, in their infinite wisdom, the wonderful benefits of incorporating pulp into other food recipes. What they fail to mention, is that laziness is not an option. In my opinion, this merely creates more work, which is the major road block why most people are lacking in their nutrition in the first place. What is the likelihood that you will actually use the pulp that way? My guess is once, maybe twice, if that. Blending is a different story.

I am not referring to your standard kitchen blender. In my experience, tossing in kale or collard greens, results in chunky, disgusting tasting drinks. Instead, you will need a powerful enough motor to liquefy these super foods. This will increase the palatability of your smoothie, and give you the infinite wisdom of what nature has to offer. Since pulp is the source of fibre, it makes no logical sense to throw away one of the absolute healthiest aspects of consuming these foods in the first place.

One of the greatest challenges in maintaining a healthy weight is overcoming sugar cravings. Foods that are broken down relatively quickly, results in elevated blood sugar along with sharp insulin spikes, which leave you craving more. Fibre dramatically helps to slow this process down so that energy levels are used in smaller amounts over longer periods of time. Why is this important? Sustained energy.[9] For this reason along with many more, fibre has been suspected of reducing development of cardiovascular disease, type 2 diabetes, and even colorectal cancer.[10]

If consumed with sufficient water, fibre expands, maintaining satiety and bulks up our stool, possibly improving constipation. Additionally, this facilitates the elimination of cholesterol, literally. Without water however, the stool can become dry and "cement-like", scraping alongside intestinal walls, causing micro abrasions and inflammation. Over time this can lead to all sorts of problems, which is why constipation may contribute to deleterious health effects that span beyond just elimination.[11,12,13] Research has pointed to food sensitivities as being a potential cause of constipation but I wonder if it may be the other way around.[14]

Hormone health, inflammation, and detoxification are maintained to large degrees through proper nutrition and elimination. While often being very nutrient dense, fibrous foods in more cases than not, happen to provide the best of both worlds[15,16] However, if you are taking medication, you should know the following. Fibre delays the time that it takes for food to travel through the digestive tract. Although this is often responsible for incredible health benefits, medication absorption may also be delayed. For that reason, always be cautious with taking any medication alongside fibre.

In addition to smoothies, there are many other fibrous rich foods. Beans, peas, chickpeas and lentils for example have not only been shown to reduce LDL cholesterol and triglycerides, but blood sugar and blood pressure lowering effects have been observed. Interestingly these are all risk factors for developing cardiovascular disease. [17] All of these factors by helping to maintain a healthy weight, can dramatically contribute to good overall cardiovascular health and good overall health in general I should add.

Although fruit provides an excellent source of fibre, I prefer not to think of this category as actual health food, but rather flavour savers. If you are like me, there is never too much of a good thing. If fruit is good, then eating copious amounts, provides even more benefit, wouldn't you agree? In case my sarcasm does not read well, in my opinion adding two fruits to a large smoothie that's shared between two or more people, is the way to go. I urge you to be careful when it comes to fruit, because they do contain sugar, natural or not, which will become stored as fat if consumed in excess.

You may have seen those advertisements that state "I would rather have 180 kcal of fruit than from one can of soft drink." I'm not arguing, as the difference is night and day, however 75 kcal for a cup of berries or a pear, can add up, especially liquefying in a blender. 1 banana (100kcal) plus a cup full of frozen blueberries is more than reasonable. If you intend to add in an apple plus some tropical frozen fruit that you found on sale, you will put yourself in a position of less caloric room for other health promoting foods such as shredded coconut, hemp hearts, or cacao nibs. Although incredibly antioxidant rich, wow do they ever contain enormous amounts of calories.

Consuming generous portions (palmful) of vegetables, notably of the green, leafy variety, is WISE™. I suggest adding just enough fruit to sway the balance of taste, in favour of igniting your buds ever so right. Over time you will find that sweeter doesn't necessarily mean tastier. 1 banana, a chunk of pineapple, or maybe 1/4-1/2 a mango are my sweeteners of choice, balancing the bitterness of greens. Is it really necessary for your smoothie to look and taste like milkshakes all the time? I mean; if you want a milkshake, there are plenty of places to get one. If you're ever in the area, Kawartha Dairy's are velvety, delicious, and loaded with sugar and fat. Chocolate is my favourite.

Organic produce is expensive and not everyone is convinced that standards are truly what certification agencies claim. Still, its undeniable that harmful sprays on our food have deleterious effects on the human body as well as our ecosystem. There are some items that are worth prioritizing, plain and simple. Organic bananas aren't that much more than the regular stuff. Apples are, however even at $8.00 for a bag of 10 medium sized organic apples, the difference is negligible. Is $0.30 extra per apple really worth the indecisiveness? Save yourself the bag of potato chips and choose organic here instead. I'm guilty of buying highly pesticide and herbicide infested produce just as much as the next North American, but a little perspective can go a long way.

Fresh, Organic, Nutrient Dense Green 'Leafies'

As you walk by the green, leafy section, you'll notice that a bushel of kale is enough to easily satisfy two-three people for a week. Even if organic is 200% the cost, in the end you are choosing to consume chemical sprays for a mere $2.00 less. Blending Organic Kale, Swiss Chard, Collard Greens are three must have organic foods that easily fit in with WISE™ philosophy. Most, if not every single risk factor for developing cardiovascular disease, benefit from these items.

There have been some concerns relating to kale's possible negative effects on thyroid health when consumed in extremely high amounts.[18] First off, the science behind this notion is very limited and old, ranging back at least until 1947 as far as I can tell, with extremely few updates. Although I don't completely disagree with the research, in my opinion, we should all be so lucky to have an overeating kale problem as the solution is simply to eat less of it. I'm infinitely more concerned with potential side effects from cholesterol-lowering Statin drugs. Lastly, unless you are an elite athlete, simply increasing physical activity gives the thyroid gland very little choice but to improve in function. If you crave fries as much as my wife or deep fried, breaded lemon chicken as much as I do, then overeating kale is the least of your problems.

Smoothies, yogurts, apple sauce, and salads are customizable and therefore perfect for adding in additional fibre, antioxidants, proteins, fats and more. In addition to be inexpensive and easy to make, I find tabouli to be bright, flavourful, and super healthy. I appreciate that some dishes should be left untouched, but why not add your own twist to an already amazing salad? Steamed broccoli, carrots, perhaps even including fresh cut chilies, only elevating this nutritional champion to another dimension.

By far, one of the most important herb in the world, is ginger. This miraculous rhizome contains at least 70+ known compounds that help our inflammatory and immune response function more optimally. Literally hundreds or more exist, which we are only beginning to understand in terms of therapeutic impact[19] Even at whopping $5.00 for a palm size piece, going organic here will place this item at the top of your inexpensive list. Try adding ginger to soups, stews, and even smoothies and you won't be sorry. Oh, it can be spicy, so a little can go a long way.

Garlic and onion are not only a staple in salads and meals for the hearty, but both have been shown to lower cholesterol in several studies. In a way, I expect most people to say "oh yeah, I love onion and garlic and add them to almost everything". In which case I hold my breath, waiting for "and yet funny enough my cholesterol is still high doc." The research is there, however using garlic and onions alongside a dollop of butter, a splash of cream, or even as part of a fatty meat dish, may not exactly fit in with what the researchers had in mind.

Of the two herbs, garlic has taken the spotlight as a supplement. In particular, aged varieties stand out as benefiting cardiovascular health. Other areas include substances within garlic, notably allicin, alliin, and others, however there has been much confusion regarding their stability in isolation. Still, there truly is nothing like crushing some raw cloves and lightly sautéing in bed of colourful veggies. Besides, the act of doing so appears to activate certain enzymes conferring greater therapeutic value.

Paying special attention to culinary herbs is by no means a waste of time. Fresh basil and oregano are favourites among creating that tomato sauce the way mama used to make. Although flavourful is an understatement, their unique healing properties have been revered throughout the ages, and modern science is slowly catching up. Sage is being studied for its anti-dementia properties. [20,21] Thyme, rosemary, and oregano are used in the preservation of supplements, notably oils. This has become innovative practice within the supplement world, notably the fish oil category, in preventing rancidity and prolonging shelf life.

With olive oil's powerful FDA approved 'lower coronary heart disease risk' claim, finding creative ways of incorporating it throughout the day makes sense. Olive oil has demonstrated a 15% reduction in LDL cholesterol, which is an incredible feat in my opinion from one food alone. [22] If that's not enough to get you oiled up, it has also been shown to increase HDL cholesterol by 5.1-6.7%. [23] Even at 240 calories, two tablespoons of EVO is negligible in the context of a large, rich, leafy, nutrient dense salad. Using a measured amount in your own personal salad dressing is a fantastic, healthier alternative to store bought versions, which often contain rancid, processed oils, emulsifiers such as EDTA, refined sugars and genetically modified, corn derivatives. Kids love colourful salads and will eat your creations up. Being creative will enable them to adjust to different flavours and let you know what they like or dislike. You may be pleasantly surprised at what they tell you.

Many within the Natural Health Industry appear fixated on discovering or creating the next best health craze. In Peru's Andes Mountains, maca root has been used for hormonal support for generations. Antioxidant rich goji and açaí berries reveal legends of unbounded energy and youthfulness from Tibet and the Amazon Rainforest, respectfully. While full credit is due for remote discoveries, it is easy to neglect those super foods that are already within our reach. Squash and parsnip are great in soups, stews, and even lightly roasted in the oven along with turnip and beet.

The positive impacts on hormone health are no strangers to the Brassica family (cruciferous) of vegetables, which include Broccoli, cauliflower, bok choy, cabbage, and Brussels sprouts. Inverse observations between consumption levels and prostate cancer, is just the tip of the iceberg. A 2011 Chinese population study involving over 134,796 adults, found these widely available masterpieces to promote cardiovascular health as well as overall longevity. [24] Mom was right; the king of all vegetables. In this way, by consuming high fibre, nutrient dense foods for the maintenance of cholesterol health, many other side benefits become your reward.

If You Must Snack at Night

Nuts are often conveniently located where the bulk candy is so my advice is not to spend too much time there. I was taught that 28 almonds per day is the daily dose by which we should consider for lowering elevated cholesterol, but many different doses have been shown to work. 66g (400kcal) of almonds, replacing 50% of a person's daily fat intake, was shown to decrease triglycerides, total cholesterol, and LDL cholesterol by 14%, 4%, and 6%, respectively, while increasing HDL by 6%.[25] 84g and 100g were also shown to have similar results. Although my wife disagrees whole heartedly, with each one weighing 1.2g, that's a lot of almonds.

I understand the addiction. You're not alone. However, you are already incorporating 2 tbsp. of EVO and 20-30g of fibre from superfood powerhouses. Therefore, 28 almonds is not only reasonable in my opinion, but fits conveniently in a 1.5ounce shot glass for measuring. Although nuts can get out of hand in terms of calories, their ability to help control appetite is impressive, leaving us feeling more than satisfied.[26] We're also less likely to scramble around for junk food. Not that we would ever dare in the first place.

Chapter 19:

Getting to the Meat

A pproaching the meat section reminds me of a great meal I had recently. Some colleagues and I each ordered a succulent, 12oz, bison steak, Delmonico, in Denver, Colorado a while back. As a 19th century reference, our server enlightened us Canadians as to the historical and marbled nature of this rather juicy preparation. While thoroughly enjoying my meal, a colleague asked me why I had trimmed off so much fat. "Saturated fat is not necessarily as bad as we once thought," she said. "Bison meat has been shown to sway our omega-3 index in favour of less inflammation, if anything," she continued. "You, of all people should know that," she finished, as her teeth sunk into that last tremendous piece like butter. In many ways, my colleague is right. Still, cooking method as well as what happens to that fat once digested, carries a lot of 'weight', regardless of what test tubes may reveal.

As I lean against the glass of the butcher's counter debating which cuts will 'meat' my fancy, I'm mindful of making

WISE™ choices. The marbled steak in Denver contained just over 200mg of cholesterol and 8g of saturated fat. Relative to an egg, these are very reasonable amounts. Adding in 1-2 whole eggs in the morning plus cream in my coffee, plus a piece of cheese on my lunch sandwich, are not. Let's just say that adding a rack of fatty ribs, or even just the skin from virtually any part of chicken meat, should be avoided.

Chicken wings are probably the absolute worst, which goes without saying. Besides their crispy, fun nature, my Dad is convinced that I'm merely addicted to the sugary sauces and insists that I "just cut up chicken breast cubes and douce them every once in a while." Although there are tasty alternative options out there such as using corn flakes as part of a baked crisp, I can't stress avoiding chicken wings and ribs enough if cholesterol levels are high. If you think deep frying renders down some fat, you are absolutely right. In your infinite wisdom however, whatever is left is highly oxidized, crisp in the first place. I'm truly in your corner on this one; just don't buy it.

Pork has been given a bad name over the years when it comes to fat, primarily because pork belly is full of it. Still, pork chops are extremely lean and provide an excellent option. A good butcher will know what the animals are being fed. If your grocery store, like one of mine, advertises "corn fed beef", I urge you to question whether you should pay their premium or run for the hills. Cows don't eat corn! Not really, anyway, and certainly not as their staple. Furthermore, consider that the corn is probably genetically modified. You may find certificates written on labels, which you can look up when you get home. Humane Certified, Organic, Free Range, are becoming more common. If you have access to the farmers themselves, then you are a step ahead of most. Not to mention, you may be able to negotiate your way into some incredible quality at superior prices.

Processed or packaged meats contain preservatives such as nitrates, which create more work for the liver. Oven roasted chicken, turkey or beef are valid cold cut options. However, eating a salad is a much healthier option than a generously stacked sandwich, wouldn't you agree? Solid, saturated fat globules should give you clues as to what a particular meat may do for cholesterol levels. In other words, don't get the spicy salami. Ironically, sausage type meats often incorporate spices, which is incredibly supportive when it comes to fat. Rosemary and thyme in particular have been shown to protect certain carcinogenic chemicals such as heterocyclic amines (HCAs) from forming during the cooking process, particularly over a flame.[1] We can certainly apply herbs to the lean stuff and in the oils that we may be heating.

The American Heart Association and World Health Organization recommends that we eat between 2-3 servings of fish per week.[2,3] However, knowing what to look for in terms of quality assurance is fishy to say the least. First, the vast majority of wild fishing areas are polluted, notably with heavy metals such as mercury, lead, and arsenic. Second, standards for sustainable fishing practices don't appear to be well laid out. In many places, wild fish are either extremely expensive or difficult to find, fresh. Farming in theory provides useful alternatives, however there are many variations in PCBs, growth hormones, and food pellets, to scratch the surface. Purchasing fish with a reputable certification agency listed on the label is a great way of investigating further on their respective websites. Ocean Wise (The Vancouver Aquarium) is one of my favourites, which is starting to make waves at specialty butcher shops. "Wild" and "Pacific" for the most part are premium options that may be worthwhile considering, otherwise.

The cheese section. Simple. Just walk on by. Seriously. Not worth it. 1 slice of cheddar contains about 30mg of cholesterol, which is certainly not the end of the world, but hefty nevertheless. Are you really going to stick with one? I'll say it again. Just walk on by.

Who Can Resist the Smell of Fresh _____?

Bread is a sensitive matter, to say the least, but I'm not referring to gluten. Truth be told, a very small percentage of people in North America have true Celiac disease. Since many of us have an emotional connection to the smell yet alone taste of freshly baked bread, I see very little reason to avoid it completely. Whole wheat as well as these new healthy grain breads that are surfacing on the market, are excellent sources of both fibre and protein (although not complete). Still, if they are so healthy, then why are most of them fortified with synthetic, vitamins and minerals? Commercial breads contain additives such as softeners, sugars, and even isolated derivatives possibly from genetically modified corn such as mono and diglycerides.

Two slices of bread are approximately 300 kcal. As a carbohydrate, eating it plain provides an incredible amount of energy without much nutrient return on your investment. Yet, most of the time we tax on copious amounts of additional condiments. Butter, highly processed margarine or mayonnaise, jam, jelly, and all sorts of spreads and sauces. I'm proposing that you choose your battle on this one. Steel cut oatmeal in the morning with cinnamon and vanilla is a great bread alternative because it acts as a vehicle for additional nutrient dense foods such as sprouted chia, flax, hemp hearts, and berries. If you must have your morning toast, I'm not judging. Perhaps forgoing a sandwich for a beautiful salad at lunch is where you'll improvise. Consider that if you don't have that loaf of bread in the house, you will have little reason to eat it. I know you love it, but there are better options.

Quinoa is a delicious option, cooked and eaten just as you would rice. Whether you prefer eating it as part of a salad, or hot, this can take the place of many other carbs while adding tremendous value in return. Unlike bread, quinoa doesn't need to be fortified with fake nutrients. Where wheat in general, falls short of a complete amino acid profile, quinoa picks up the slack offering the real McCoy. Many books have been written regarding the health benefits of magnesium alone and quinoa provides an outstanding source, as do hemp hearts by the way.

Sprouted brown rice in addition to being a great fibre source, is loaded with naturally occurring B vitamins as well as gamma-aminobutyric acid (GABA). You may recognize this substance in the supplement world as a naturally occurring neurotransmitter in the brain, which is highly involved in us maintaining our cool, calm, collected state of mind. For that reason it's often used therapeutically to treat conditions such as anxiety and depression. [4] An enzyme called GABA-t (transaminase) breaks down our beloved hero, which can be disrupting to say the least. One herb called Melissa officinalis (Lemon Balm) has been shown to inhibit this enzyme thus helping to maintain and even possibly elevating GABA. [5] Lemon balm is generally regarded as safe and interestingly enough promotes focus at low dosages, yet sleep at higher amounts, among other fabulous side benefits. By sprouting the rice, enzymes are released and antioxidants are further enhanced. Replacing wheat with sprouted brown rice, therefore provides excellent long term return on your caloric investment.

Other amazing, nutrient dense grains include amaranth, buckwheat, and spelt, to name a few. These, in addition to certain dairy products, oatmeal, and unsweetened apple sauces, are fantastic vehicles for nutritional add-ons. We already mentioned some oatmeals add-ons, but the point I'm trying to make, is customization. If convenience overrules and you prefer flash freeze dried berries, greens, or protein powders, there's very little stopping you from adding them in here. Hemp hearts or even hemp protein powders are among my favourites. Sprouted, organic chia seeds are loaded with antioxidants and omega 3 fatty acids and are primarily a source of insoluble fibre. Sprouted, organic flax seeds have similar benefits yet offers a mix of almost half and half soluble and insoluble.

Protein rich Greek or Icelandic yogurt, and cottage cheeses are fantastic dairy options to place in your basket. In addition to offering a wide array of minerals including calcium and magnesium, 5-10mg of cholesterol per serving is very low. Even at 25mg, a measuring cup will easily keep you on track. Being aware of serving size is one of the greatest tips I can offer with respect to food label reading of any kind. This is how you will make the most out of reading Fibre, protein, fat, and sugar content before jotting on your list.

Our bodies run on protein. Enzymes? Protein. Collagen for hair, skin, and nail health? Protein. Muscle growth and function? You guessed it. Mental wellbeing? I see little reason to look at any other supplement on the market if protein intake isn't up to par. How much are you receiving, relative to what your body needs? An average, athletic person needs about 0.8g for every kilogram that they weigh (2.2 pounds for every kg). If you weigh 150 pounds, divide it by 2.2 to get roughly 68.2kg. Then multiply that by 0.8 to get your daily protein requirement which in this case is 54.5g. One medium sized chicken breast offers about 23g and a serving of Greek yogurt, 16g. Quinoa contains protein as does the egg you had for breakfast (about 6g per egg white).

More often than not, there should be very little reason to go into the packaged goods isles of a grocery store. Still, here is what I look for on packaged goods' labels. For the most part realizing that mono and diglycerides, and maltodextrin, pretty much all come from corn. They are highly processed using harsh chemicals. Moreover, they probably come from GMO corn. The same holds true for corn starches and syrups. Lastly, trans fat should always be zero or say "trans-fat free." Non-GMO Verification Project's seal is the best way to know whether your purchase is indeed GMO or not. Although organic certification agencies do not allow GMO products, they do not possess third party testing methods to verify.

Other ingredients to avoid, include colourings, MSG (monosodium glutamate) and other preservatives, soy oil, and soy derivatives such lecithin, which are also likely GMO, and highly processed using harsh chemicals and heat. If you don't know what an ingredient is, don't buy the food. In general, I find that products which contain trans-fat, corn, and soy derivatives, also include anything else that you can imagine. For that reason, there's not much point in looking any further. I promise that you will have difficult enough time trying to find packaged goods free of the aforementioned.

I applaud the savvy shopper who vote with their dollars, choosing Non-GMO Verified and Certified Organic, packaged goods. There are some great products out there, made with simple ingredients, which grandma would approve. Nevertheless, I propose that sugar be placed into context. 5g-10g of fibre per serving is outstanding on a label, however if sugar is one of the main ingredients, consider putting it down and grabbing a can of beans instead. Sugar means extra calories plus a reduction in the same level of sustained energy that you will receive from the simple stuff already in your cart. That delicious green smoothie is calling your name.

Before heading to the checkouts, certain canned foods as well as the freezer section is worth considering. Of course I'm not referring to prepared food, but rather produce. Although counterintuitive, both canned as well as frozen items are often packaged in peak season and optimal environments. Tomatoes provide a fantastic example. With the exception of maybe a month or so in the fall, I find our tomatoes Ontario absolutely flavourless. Most of the time they're imported from Mexico and ripen on transport. Widely available, Italian, canned tomatoes on the other hand, are incredibly sweet and juicy, ripened and picked in their prime.

My kids and I love blueberries, either on their own as a snack or as part of a green smoothie. The fresh versions in the produce section look like mutant berries. They're huge and I just don't trust them. Wild berries are of course much smaller and found, well, in the wild. Certified organic or certified pesticide free varieties are absolutely delicious, and available all year round thanks to flash freezing technologies. Price points are lower than fresh and although not everyone will agree, from my experience, quality may be just as good or dare I say much better. Lastly, if you do happen to have left over fresh fruit or vegetables, placing them in airlock bags and into the freezer is an excellent way to prevent spoilage.

Chapter 20:

The Forbidden Fruit

Having stemmed from a science background, my naturopathic studies were initiated through a fascination with herbs and supplements. I was enamored with their pharmaceutical-like properties. Evaluating mechanism of action and adverse reactions felt as though we were learning about 'real' medicine; the medicine of the future. However, in light of what we've discussed with respect to nutraceutical processing, I must admit; complexity, synergy, and safety, have become front of mind. Holism, rather than reductionistic fractions, provide the best of what nature has to offer.

I have shared my views on cholesterol, heart disease, and the aging process, rethinking chronic disease as we know it. Major root causes stem from our body's failed attempt at optimally improving its immune and stress response, oxidative defense mechanisms, and metabolic distribution and usage of energy. It was my intention to stress the importance of creating an environment where cholesterol (and thus our cells) can thrive as optimally as possible in the face of these aforementioned challenges. Simply put, protecting while being moderate of energy consumption and usage; the forbidden fruit in my opinion. Furthermore, I'm grateful for the opportunity to share my method of diet diary analysis, to serve as a useful tool along your journey towards promoting lifelong wellness. Lastly, I hope to have decluttered the confusing and often intimidating jungle of expanding information, contained within the natural health industry and naturopathic medical profession, in a way that you, the layperson, receives tremendous value from.

After providing you with my grocery store walk through however, I find myself torn. The purpose of this book is to share with you my absolute best. Without a doubt, whole food is it. Not to mention, supplements and herbs almost sounds like a recipe for another book in of itself. Some more than others however, have incredible merit in discussing further with your doctor and I'll take a moment here to share with you some great examples.

Plant sterols have been so well researched that Health Canada has written a report revealing that an 8.8% drop LDL-Cholesterol has been observed with a dosage of merely 2g per day. This is while having no known negative effects on HDL, resulting in an overall improvement in a person's lipid profile if they have been diagnosed with having moderately high cholesterol.[1] The proposed mechanism of action is by blocking the absorption of cholesterol from the digestive tract.[2] Many supplement companies have now marketed the use of these substances, most notably under the names beta-sitosterols, stigmasterols, campesterols, beta-sterolins.

In my experience, soy is often used as a source of plant sterols, so looking for key quality distinctions is a good idea, as opinions regarding soy are controversial to say the least. The Non-GMO Project Verification seal highlights a mark of reassurance, in my opinion. Also, as oils are at risk of rancidity, antioxidants listed on the label such as green tea extract, rosemary, oregano, may help. Requesting a rancimat score from a company or inquiring about product stability, is an excellent way to investigate for yourself as well. Some food for thought; nutrient dense whole fruits and vegetables, nuts, and seeds, already naturally contain plant sterols.

Niacin or B3, has profound cholesterol lowering properties, which are recognized by some of the most renown medical institutions around the world.[3] I'd like to caution you however regarding a side effect or benefit (whichever way you look at it) of "flushing". Niacin causes inflammatory prostaglandins to be released called D2. For my third year naturopathic nutrition exam, I purposely took enough niacin to cause a flush for the duration of the exam. My face turned lobster red and my ears were tingling almost to the point of burning. It feels like a sunburn underneath the skin and although goes away naturally, was extremely uncomfortable as you might imagine. You might be interested to know that by continuously causing the flush, the body ends up depleting itself of prostaglandin D2 and so flushing is actually its own antidote in a way. Although niacin is not a favourite of mine for this reason, the science behind it is simply too great to ignore and so I'm including it for your consideration.

High quality fish oils are more than worthwhile. Fresh varieties are hard to come by, at least in Ontario. Supplementing makes a lot of sense in my opinion. Here is what I look for. Ocean Wise certified, Non-GMO Project Verified, extra virgin, and wild. Products, which provide 2-3 servings of fish per week satisfy the American Heart Association and World Health Organization's serving recommendations. Clinical trials and third party testing for heavy metals and dioxins are worth asking for as well.

The liver produces cholesterol. Implementing protective strategies, is therefore best practice. With no shortages in choice, very few herbs in my mind stand out as much as turmeric, artichoke, dandelion root, milk thistle, and of course ginger. Many high quality detoxification formulas include these as their main ingredients. However, by empowering yourself and your family to insist on WISE™ dietary and lifestyle choices, the liver naturally becomes properly nourished, while being less taxed in my opinion. Most 'detoxes in a box' fail to provide protein and fibre, which are the absolute essential aspects of elimination, both from a physical and physiological point of view. Adding in some Greek yogurt and a tbsp. of sprouted, organic chia or flax seeds can go a long way even on a calorie restricted cleanse/diet. The same holds true for a hemp heart, green smoothie. Speak with your doctor about what may be right for you.

Lowering elevated cholesterol is easy. We have pharmaceutical drugs for that. Still, they are certainly not free from side effects and fail to address the major root causes of cardiovascular disease and chronic disease risk in the first place. Where natural medicines may fall short in areas where drugs excel, such as in their ability to control biochemical rate limiting steps, long term safety as well as complexity are certainly a strength worth valuing, offering incredible bonus side benefits. Reducing abnormally elevated cholesterol is important, but cholesterol in general can be used as a wonderful model in my opinion to explain chronic disease risk as well as propose preventative and treatment strategies, helping to promote lifelong wellness.

For a certain portion of our lives, the human body appears capable of repairing damage more efficiently than accruing, which is of course evidenced partially by the fact that we grow and mature in the first place. Eventually however, constant bombardment catches up, resulting in the form of aging and age related chronic diseases. Cardiovascular disease is perhaps the most well-known and well-studied. Could fasting reveal answers? A recent study out of the university of Southern California certainly caught my attention, which demonstrated that people who were undergoing chemotherapy to treat certain forms of cancer, when fasting for 3-5 days, regenerated certain aspects of their immune system.[4] Nutrition provides us with the means to exist, yet ironically and most notably food energy sources, may contribute to our very demise.

Although I'm not a religious man, in Judaism, the Jewish People fast on Yom Kippur to atone for their sins. As well, The Torah writes of the sin of eating the forbidden fruit, ridding humanity of our once supposed immortality/extremely long lifespans. Can a connection be made between atoning for sin by restricting food intake, with fruit, and with lifespan; perhaps an ancient clue, outside of modern day science? Is energy from food the forbidden fruit, and if so, how do we protect ourselves, or rather protect the energy itself from forming into its worst versions for human health? An apple turns brown, sugar caramelizes, meat burns. Spices, cooking methods, stress and inflammatory processes within the body can alter these processes and how they interact with our physiology and development of chronic disease as well as the aging process.

Fermented food is particularly interesting in terms of a protective 'food group' for immune, inflammatory, and oxidative changes within our food and bodies. As a staple of humanity, and with thousands of published articles, we have barely scratch the surface in our understanding with respect to fermentation and human health. Possibly millions of ferment metabolites and unique bacteriocins, exist within brines or 'mediums' in foods such as yogurt and kefir. Raw food is healthy, yet fermenting the same food provides a nourishment which is infinitely more complex. Reducing allergens and enzyme inhibitors, miraculously allows us to obtain more out fermented versions. They are truly beyond raw, yet not cooked. Cabbage and tofu may be difficult to digest raw, but miso, tempeh, sauerkraut, and kimchi, go down easy while contributing greatly towards improving digestive health. A sort of alchemy indeed, where synergy of nutrients provide mathematics where 2 plus 2 equals ten thousand plus. Perhaps our answers don't exist solely within nutrition itself, but within the innate intelligence of the microbial world, implanted onto the foods that we thrive on. Maybe the rest of the animal kingdom knows something that we humans, with all our technology, are just at the brink of discovering, that may change everything.

I find it fascinating that soy's phytoestrogen content sparks controversy at every turn. Soy contains molecules which look like estrogen, and can influence the way different versions of estrogen work in the body, by influencing their receptor sites, essentially. Although many companies promote soy as a wonder food for hormonal health, there is controversy around increased potential cancer risk associated with consuming too much soy, especially with respect to estrogen sensitive cancers such as breast and uterine. In my opinion, context and moderation needs to be taken into consideration here as well as distinctions such as whether the soy consumed has been genetically modified and contains dangerous chemicals used in its mass farming around the world. By fermenting soy and creating say tempeh, the soy becomes transformed into almost a completely different food, with its phytoestrogens or isoflavones as they are called, changing in both structure and function. Genestein changes into Genestin, and so forth, dramatically telling a different story within modern literature pertaining to cancer risk and prevention.

As a general rule, I may include minute amounts of soy in my diet such as those little pieces of tofu found in 'restaurant' miso soup, and prefer to consumer more moderate (but not extreme) amounts of fermented soy such as the miso itself, and tempeh. By the way, where many people use unfermented soy, such as tofu, as a plant based protein source, my personal feeling is that switching to a more nutrient dense, pre-digested, transformed, fermented version such as tempeh, is a much better route to take.

I want to take this opportunity to congratulate you in taking your health seriously and thank you for allowing me to share some of my best information, which I have and continue to dedicate my life's work towards. Asking ourselves how we can reach our greatest potentials, begins with imagination, yet leans on knowledge. By improving and extending your quality of life, working towards being your best self is not only inspiring, but I promise you that it is infectious. There's a saying where people wish onto others to 'live until 120'. I wish you and your family lifelong wellness, far beyond.

With Sincerest Gratitude,

Dr. Robert W. Horovitz, B.Sc., ND

References

Prelude

[1] The top 10 Causes of death. World Health Organization. Fact sheet N°310. Updated May, 2014. Accessed Oct. 2014. http://www.who.int/mediacentre/factsheets/fs310/en/

Introduction

[1] Wine RX. 60 Minutes Interview. Dr. David Sinclair, Harvard University. Produced by Deirdre Naphil Curran, Kathy Textor.

[2] Guarente, L. Sirtuins in Aging and Disease. CSH Symposia on Quantitiative Biology. 2007 72: 483-488. Cold Springs Harbor Press. Accessed December 1, 2014.

[3] Kaeberlein, Matt et al. Substrate-specific Activation of Sirtuins by Resveratrol. The Journal of Biological Chemistry. Vol. 280, No. 17, Issue of April 20, pp.17038-17045, 2005. Web. 1 Dec. 2014.

[4] Baur, Joseph A et al. Resveratrol improves health and survival of mice on a high-caloric diet. Nature Publishing Group. Vol 444. 16 November 2006. Doi:10.1038. Web. 1 Dec. 2014.

[5] David Sinclair Bio. Ted Med 2014. Speakers: David Sinclair. www.tedmed.com/speakers/show?id=6542. Web. 1 Dec. 2014.

[6] Farombi, E. O. & Onyema, O. O. (2006). "Monosodium Glutamate-Induced Oxidative Damage and Genotoxicity in the Rat: Modulatory Role of Vitamin C, Vitamin E and Quercetin," Hum Exp Toxicol, 25(5), 251-9.

[7] Veronika Husarova and Daniela Ostatnikova (2013), "Monosodium Glutamate Toxic Effects and Their Implications for Human Intake: A Review," JMED Research, Vol. 2013 (2013), Article ID 608765, DOI: 10.5171/2013.608765

[8] Padayaty, J Sebastian et al. Human adrenal glands secrete vitamin C in response to adrenocorticotrophic hormone. American Journal of Clinical Nutrition. 2007; 86: 145-9.

[9] Prousky JE. The Orthomolecular Treatment of Schizophrenia: A Primer for Clinicians. Townsend Letter. Best of Naturopathic Medicine. February/March 2007: 90.

[10] Smythies JR. The role of ascorbate in brain: Therapeutic implications. J R Soc Med, i996:89:24I

[11] Sharma SR, et al. Effect of vitamin C on collagen biosynthesis and degree of birefringence in polarization sensitive optical coherence tomography (PS-OCT). African Journal of Biotechnology Vol. 7(12), pp. 2049-2054, 17 June, 2008.

[12] Clark, Kristine L. Nutritional Considerations in Joint Health. Clinics In Sports Medicine. 26 (2007) 106. Elsevier Inc, 2007.

[13] Park, Seyeon. The Effects of High Concentrations of Vitamin C on Cancer Cells. Review. Nutrients. 2013, 5, 3496; dii: 10.3390/nu5093496

[14] Kamel NS, et al. Antioxidants and hormones as antiaging therapies: High hopes, disappointing results. Review: Cleveland Clinic Journal of Medicine. Volume 73, Number 12. 2006: 1049-1056.

[15] Belcaro G, et al. Improvement in signs and symptoms in psoriasis patients with Pycnogenol® supplementation. Panminerva Medica 2014 March; 56(1):41-8.

[16] Mala Jr H, et al. Combining oral contraceptives with a natural nuclear factor-kappa B inhibitor for the treatment of endometriosis-related pain. International Journal of Women's Health. 2014:6 35-39.

[17] Huangfu J, et al. Antiaging effects of astaxanthin-rich alga Haematococcus pluvialis on fruit flies under oxidative stress. Journal of Agricultural and Food Chemistry. 2013, 61 (32), pp 7800-7804.

[18] Wu W, et al. Astaxanthin alleviates brain aging in rats by attenuating oxidative stress and increasing BDNF levels. Food and Function. 2014, 5, 158-166.

[19] Yoon HS. , Cho Hyun Hee, Cho Soyun, Lee Se-Rah, Shin Mi-Hee, and Chung Jin Ho. Journal of Medicinal Food. July 2014, 17(7): 810-816. doi:10.1089/jmf.2013.3060.

[20] Katagiri, Mikiyuki et al. Effects of astaxanthin-rich Haematococcus pluvialis extract on cognitive function: a randomised, double-blind, placebo-controlled study. Journal of Clinical Biochemistry Nutrition. September 2012, Volum 51, Number 2. 102-107.

[21] T.M. Brasky, C. et al. Serum Phospholipid Fatty Acids and Prostate Cancer Risk: Results From the Prostate Cancer Prevention Trial. American Journal of Epidemiology, 2011; 173 (12): 1429 DOI: 10. 1093/ajekwr027.

[22] A tide of evidence washes away flawed fish oil prostate cancer study. Alliance for Natural Health: Europe. Web. Dec. 2, 2014. http://anh-europe.org/news/a-tide-of-evidence-washes-away-flawed-fish-oil-prostate-cancer-study.

[23] Ferrieres, Jean. The French Paradox: Lessons for Other Countries. Heart. Coronary Disease. 2004; 90: 107-111.

Ferrieres, Jean. The French Paradox: Lessons for Other Countries. Heart. Coronary Disease. 2004; 90: 107-111.

eins (sirtuins) metabolize NAD and may have protein ADP-ribosyltransferase activity". Biochemical and Biophysical Research Communications. Volume 260 (1): 273–9. doi:10.1006/bbrc.1999.0897

[25] Hooper Judith. Of Moths and Men: An Evolutionary Tale: the Untold Story of Science and the Peppered Moth. Norton, 2002.

[26] What is a gene. Genetics Home Reference: Your Guide to Understanding Genetic Conditions. Web. Dec. 1, 2014. http://ghr.nlm.nih.gov/handbook/basics/gene.

[27] Fu, Li, et al. Effects of high-fat diet and regular aerobic exercise on global gene expression in skeletal muscle of C57BL/6 mice. Metabolism Clinical and Experimental. 61 (2012). pp.146–152.

[28] Davies, Kelvin JA. Oxidative Stress, Antioxidant Defenses, and Damage Removal, Repair, and Replacement Systems. IUBMB Life, 50: 279-289, 2000.

[29] Lakatta EG. Age-associated cardiovascular changes in health: impact on cardiovascular disease in older persons. Heart Fail Rev. 2002 Jan;7(1):29-49.

[30] Bianconi, Eva et al. An estimation of the number of cells in the human body. Annals of Human Biology. 5 July 2013; Early Online: 1-11. Web. 2 Dec 2014.

[31] Asimuddin M, Jamil K. Insight into the DNA repair mechanism operating during cell cycle checkpoints in eukaryotic cells. Review Article. Biology and Medicine, 4 (4): 147-166, 2012.

[32] Molgora Brenda, et al. Functional Assessment of Pharmacological Telomerase Activators in Human T Cells. Cells 2013, 2, 57-66; dii: 10.3390/cells2010057.

[33] Harley, Calvin B. A Natural Product Telomerase Activator As Part of a Health Maintenance Program. Rejuvenation Research. Volume 14, Number 1, 2011. Mary Ann Liebert, Inc. DOI: 10.1089/rej.2010.1085.

CHAPTER 1

[1] Metabolic pathways — Reference pathway. KEGG; Kanehisa Laboratories. 1005-2014. Web. Dec. 4, 2014. http://goo.gl/GIhCNX

[2] Part 1: Metabolic Pathways. Hoffmann-La Roche Ltd. 2014. Web. 3 Dec 2014. http://biochemical-pathways.com/#/map/1.

[3] Boothe, DM. Imidazoles. The Merck Veterinary Manual. March, 2012. Web. 3 Dec 2014. http://www.merckmanuals.com/vet/pharmacology/antifungal_agents/imidazoles.html. face

[4] Alberts, B. The Lipid Bilayer. Molecular Biology of the Cell. 4th Edition. Garland Science. 2002. Web. 3 Dec 2014. http://www.ncbi.nlm.nih.gov/books/NBK26871/.

[5] Definition: Blockbuster Drug. Investopedia. Web. 3 Dec 2014. http://www.investopedia.com/terms/b/blockbuster-drug.asp.

[6] Thompson, Gilbert R. Absorption of fat-soluble vitamins and sterols. J.clin.Path.,24,Suppl.(Roy.Coll.Path.),5,85-89.

[7] Miller, Walter L et al. Ovarian and Adrenal Androgen Biosynthesis and Metabolism. Contemp Endo: Androgen Excess Disorders in Women PCOS and Other Disorders, 2nd Ed. Humana Press. 2007.

[8] Miller WL. Molecular biology of steroid hormone synthesis. Endocr Rev 1988;9:295–318.

[9] Sanderson, Thomas J. The Steroid Hormone Biosynthesis Pathway as a Target for Endocrine-Disrupting Chemicals: Review. Toxicological Sciences: 94(1), 3–21 (2006) doi:10.1093/toxsci/kfl051

CHAPTER 2

[1] Singh, Parminder. Andropause: Current Concepts: Review. Indian Journal of Endocrinology and Metabolism. 2013. Vol 17. Supplement 3.
[2] Mayo Clinic Staff. Diseases and Conditions: Menopause. 1998-2014. Web. 3 Dec 2014.
http://www.mayoclinic.org/diseases-conditions/menopause/basics/definition/con-20019726.
[3] Morgentaler, Abraham. Testosterone Replacement Therapy and Prostate Cancer. Urol Clin N Am 34 (2007) 555–563.
[4] Morgentaler, Abraham. New Concepts Regarding Testosterone and Prostate Cancer: A Breath of Fresh Air. Oncology Journal, Genitourinary Cancers, Prostate Cancer. May 15, 2014. UBM Medica, Web. 5 Dec 2014.
http://goo.gl/pFtHge.
[5] Definition @ Merriam-Webster online: -sterone
[6] Funder JW, Krozowski Z, Myles K, Sato A, Sheppard KE, Young M (1997). "Mineralocorticoid receptors, salt, and hypertension". *Recent Prog Horm Res* 52: 247–260. PMID 9238855
[7] Gupta BBP, Lalchhandama K (2002). "Molecular mechanisms of glucocorticoid action". *Current Science* **83** (9): 1103–1111.
[8] Frye CA (2009). "Steroids, reproductive endocrine function, and affect. A review". *Minerva Ginecol* 61 (6): 541–562. PMID 19942840
[9] Miller, Walter L et al. Ovarian and Adrenal Androgen Biosynthesis and Metabolism. Contemp Endo: Androgen Excess Disorders in Women PCOS and Other Disorders, 2nd Ed. Humana Press. 2007.
[10] Fiore, Robert and Butler, George. Pumping Iron. White Mountain Films. 1977.
[11] Schoenfeld, Brad J. The Mechanisms of Muscle Hypertrophy and Their Application to Resistance Training. Journal of Strength & Conditioning Res. 24(10)/2857–2872.
[12] Tim Muriello Rich Piana Converssations Part 2: High Reps VS Heavy Weight. I'llPumpYouUp.com. YouTube Published Jan. 10, 2014.
https://www.youtube.com/watch?v=Gi6R3e6KlTc.
[13] Bender, David A. Amino Acid Metabolism: Arginine, Cirtulline and Ornithine. John Wiley & Sons, Ltd. 2012: 209-218.
[14] Derave W, Ozdemir MS, Harris R, Pottier A, Reyngoudt H, Koppo K, Wise JA, Achten E. (August 9, 2007). "Beta-alanine supplementation augments muscle carnosine content and attenuates fatigue during repeated isokinetic contraction bouts in trained sprinters". J Appl Physiol 103 (5): 1736–43. doi:10.1152/japplphysiol.00397.2007.

0

[15] Hill CA, Harris RC, Kim HJ, Harris BD, Sale C, Boobis LH, Kim CK, Wise JA. (2007). "Influence of beta-alanine supplementation on skeletal muscle carnosine concentrations and high intensity cycling capacity". Amino Acids 32 (2): 225–33. doi:10.1007/s00726-006-0364-4.

[16] Elaki, Ramin K et al. Study on the Effects of Various Doses of Tribulus Terristris Extract on Epididymal Sperm Morphology and Count in Rat. Global Veterinaria 10 (1): 13-17, 2013. DOI: 10.5829/idosi.gv.2013.10.1.7158.

[17] Janer-Gual G. Steroid Levels, Steroid Metabolic Pathways and Their Modulation by Endocrine Disruptors In Invertebrates. Universitat Autonoma de Barcelona. Programa de Doctorat de Famacologia Terapeutica, Toxicologia. 2005; 39.

CHAPTER 3

[1] Dog, Tieraona L. Menopause: a review of botanical dietary supplements. The American Journal of Medicine (2005) Vol 118 (12B), 98S–108S

[2] Mahady GB. Is black cohosh estrogenic? *Nutr Rev.* 2003;61(pt 1): 183–186.

[3] Vitex agnus-castus. Alternative Medicine Review. Vol. 14, No 1. 2009.

[4] Vegeto, E et al. Estrogen and inflammation: hormone generous action spreads to the brain. Molecular Psychiatry. 2002, Volume 7, Number 3, Pages 236-238.

[5] Bechlioulis, A et al. Increased vascular inflammation in early menopausal women is associated with hot flush severity. J Clin Endocrinol Metab. 2012 May;97(5):E760-4. doi: 10.1210/jc.2011-3151.

[6] Locative, Sampaio GP and Fleiuss de Farias, ML. Osteoporosis and Inflammation: Review. Arq Bras Endocrinol Metab. 2010;54/2.

[7] Osteoporosos. University of Maryland Medical Centre. Reviewed: 12/19/2012. Web. 5 Dec 2014. http://umm.edu/health/medical/reports/articles/osteoporosis

[8] Cilotti, Antonio and Falchetti, Alberto. Clinical Cases in Mineral and Bone Metabolism 2009; 6(3): 229-233.

[9] Ciapauch, Ruth. Total estradiol, rather than testosterone levels, predicts osteoporosis in aging men. Arq Bras Endocrinol Metab. 2009;53/8.

[10] Gual GJ. Steroid Levels, Steroid Metabolic Pathways and Their Modulation by Endocrine Disruptors In Invertebrates. Universitat Autonoma de Barcelona. Programa de Doctorat de Famacologia Terapeutica, Toxicologia. 2005; 34.

[11] Kiecolt-Glaser, Janice K. Chronic stress and age related increases in the pro-inflammatory cytokine IL-6. PNAS. July 22, 2003: Vol 100, No. 15. 9090-9095.

[12] Payne, Anita H and Hales, Dale B. Overview of Steroidogenic Enzymes in the Pathway from Cholesterol to Active Steroid Hormones. Endocrine Reviews, December 2004, 25(6):947–970.

[13] Straub, Rainer H et al. Anti-inflammatory cooperativity of corticosteroids and norepinephrine in rheumatoid arthritis synovial tissue in vivo and vitro. FASEB J. 2002 Jul;16(9):993-1000.

[14] Adrenal Function Panel. Rocky Mountain Analytical. www.rmalab/node/41. Web. Feb. 6, 2016.

[15] Corbett, BA et al. Examining cortisol rhythmicity and responsivity to stress in children with Tourette syndrome. Psychoneuroendocrinology (2008) 33, 810-820.

CHAPTER 4

[1] Russel, Fiona M. Evidence on the use of paracetamol in febrile children. Bulletin of the World Health Organization 2003;81:367-372.

[2] Rosenspire, Allen J. Cutting Edge: Fever-Associated Temperatures Enhance Neutrophil Responses to Lipopolysaccharide: A Potential Mechanism Involving Cell Metabolism. J Immunol 2002; 169:5396-5400; doi: 10.4049.

[3] Nesse, Randolph M and Young, Elizabeth A. Evolutionary Origins and Functions of the Stress Response. Encyclopedia of Stress. Volume 2. 2000. 79-84.

[4] Nippoldt, Todd B. Is there such a thing as adrenal fatigue? Mayo Clinic: Diseases & Conditions - Addison's Disease. Web. 7 Dec 2014. http://goo.gl/wYsBG6.

[5] Langsjoen, Peter H. The clinical use of HMG CoA-reducatase inhibitors (statins) and the associated depletion of the essential co-factor coenzyme Q10: a review of pertinent human and animal data. Web. 5 Dec 2014. http://www.fda.gov/ohrms/dockets/dailys/02/May02/052902/02p-0244-cp00001-02-Exhibit_A-vol1.pdf.

[6] Kettawan, Aikkarach et al. Protective Effects of Coenzyme Q10 on Decreased Oxidative Stress Resistance Induced by Simvastatin. J. Clin. Biochem. Nutr., 40, 194–202, May 2007

[7] Mancuso, Michelangelo et al. Coenzyme Q10 and Neurological Diseases: Review. Pharmaceuticals 2009, 2, 134-149; doi:10.3390/ph203134.

CHAPTER 5

[1] Understand Your Risk of Heart Attack. The American Heart Association; Oct 27, 2014. Web. 8 Dec 2014. http://goo.gl/vRTv3i.

[2] Elizabeth Holmes. TedMed 2014. Web. 8 Dec 2014. http://www.tedmed.com/speakers/show?id=308981

[3] Crane, Rachel. She's America's youngest female billionaire - and a dropout. CNN Money - Innovation Nation. October 16, 2014. Web. 8 Dec 2014. http://goo.gl/ZoGHws.

[4] Cholesterol - what you can do to lower your level. 2007 rev. The College of Family Physicians of Canada. Web. 8 Dec 2014.

CHAPTER 7

[1] Assies J et al. Effects of oxidative stress on fatty acid and one-carbon-metabolism in psychiatric and cardiovascular disease comorbidity. Acta Psychiatr Scand 2014: 130: 163–180. DOI: 10.1111/acps.12265.

[2] Tomkin, Gerald H and Owens Daphne. LDL as a Cause of Atherosclerosis. The Open Atherosclerosis & Thrombosis Journal, 2012, 5, 13-21.

[3] Spagnoli, LG et al. Role of Inflammation in Atherosclerosis. J Nucl Med 2007; 48:1800–1815
DOI: 10.2967/jnumed.107.038661.

[4] Fats and Cholesterol: Out with the Bad, In with the Good. Harvard School of Public Health. Web. 8 Dec 2014.
http://www.hsph.harvard.edu/nutritionsource/fats-full-story/.

[5] Siri-Tarino, PW et al. Saturated fat, carbohydrates, and cardiovascular disease. Am J Clin Nutr 2010;91:502–9.

CHAPTER 8

[1] Kanner J. Dietary advanced lipid per oxidation end products are risk factors to human health. Mol Nutr Food Res. 2007 Sep;51(9): 1094-101.

[2] Warnakulasuriya, Sumudu N et al. Long Chain Fatty Acid Acylated Derivatives of Quercetin-3-0-Gucoside as Antioxidants to Prevent Lipid Oxidation. Biomolecules 2014, 4, 980-993; doi:10.3390/biom4040980.

[3] Blaylock, Russell L. Excitotoxicity: A Possible Central Mechanism in Fluoride Neurotoxicity. Fluoride 2004; 37(4): 301-314 Research Review 301.

[4] Perfluorinated Chemicals (PFCs). National Institute of Environmental Health Sciences. National Institutes of Health. September 12. Web. Dec. 2, 2014.
https://www.niehs.nih.gov/health/materials/perflourinated_chemicals_508.pdf.

[5] Klausner, Victor B. Nutritional Impact on Lipid Oxidation and Coronary Artery Disease. Hospital Physician. July, 1999: 27-38.

[6] WHO. Guideline: Sodium intake for adults and children. Geneva, World Health Organization (WHO), 2012. Web. Dec. 2, 2014.
http://www.who.int/nutrition/publications/guidelines/sodium_intake_printversion.pdf

CHAPTER 9

[1] How to Taste Olive Oil. Olive Oil Times Feature: All About Olive Oil. Web. Dec. 2, 2014. www.oliveoiltimes.com/olive-oil.
[2] Boskou, Dimitrios. Olive Oil Chemistry and Technology: Storage and Packing. Laboratory of Food and Chem and Tech School of Chem, Aristotle University. Greece. AOCS Press. 2006. Web. Dec. 2, 2014.
[3] Heart & Vascular Team. Heart-Healthy Cooking: Oils 101. Cleveland Clinic. October 1, 2014. Web. Dec. 2, 2014. http://health.clevelandclinic.org/2014/10/heart-healthy-cooking-oils-101/
[4] Enos WF, Beyer J, Holmes RH. Pathogenesis of coronary disease in American soldiers killed in Korea. JAMA. 1955; 158 (11): 912-914.
[5] Joseph, Abraham et al. Manifestations of Coronary Atherosclerosis in Young Trauma Victims — An Autopsy Study. Journal of the American College of Cardiology. Vol. 22, No. 2. August, 1993: 459-67.
[6] Psaltopoulou, Theodora. Olive oil, the Mediterranean diet, and arterial blood pressure: the Greek European Prospective Investigation into Cancer and Nutrition (EPIC) study 1, 2, 3.Am J Clin Nutr October 2004 vol. 80 no. 4 1012-1018.
[7] Wahrburg, Ursel et al. Mediterranean diet, olive oil and health. Eur. J. Lipid Sci. Technol. 104 (2002) 698–705.
[8] Perfluorinated Chemicals (PFCs). National Institute of Environmental Health Sciences. National Institutes of Health. September 12. Web. Dec. 2, 2014. https://www.niehs.nih.gov/health/materials/perflourinated_chemicals_508.pdf
[9] Munn, Kevin, Borkey, Peter. Overview of Perfluorinated Chemicals (PFCs) and Related International Initiatives. United Nations Environmental Programme (UNEP) and Organization for Economic Co-operation and Development (OECD). Web. Dec. 2, 2014.http://www.oecd.org/ehs/pfc/48609862.pdf.

CHAPTER 10

[1] Labban, Louay. Medicinal and pharmacological properties of Turmeric (Curcuma long): a review. Int J Pharm Biomed Sci. 2014;5(1):17-23. ISSN No: 0976-5263.
[2] Extracts, Standardized. Jonas: Mosby's Dictionary of Complementary and Alternative Medicine. 2005. Elsevier. Web. 2 Dec 2014. http://medical-dictionary.thefreedictionary.com/extracts.
[3] Bode-Boger, Stefanie M et al. L-Argininge Induces Nitric Oxide-Dependent Vasodilation in Patients With Critical Limb Ischemia: A Randomized, Controlled Study. Circulation. 1996; 93: 85-90. Doi: 10. 1161/01.CIR.93.1.85.

[4] Pearce, Frederick L et al. Mucosal Mast Cells: III. Effect of quercetin and other flavonoids on antigen-induced histamine secretion from rat intestinal mast cells. Journal of Allergy and Clinical Immunology. Vol 73, Issue 6: 819-823. June 1984.

[5] Bucca, C. et al. Effects of Vitamin C on airway responsiveness to inhaled histamine in heavy smokers. Eur Respir J. 1989, 2, 229-233.

[6] Kettawan, Aikkarach et al. Protective Effects of Coenzyme Q10 on Decreased Oxidative Stress Resistance Induced by Simvastatin. J. Clin. Biochem. Nutr., 40, 194–202, May 2007

[7] Lee, Duk-Hee. Does supplemental vitamin C increase cardiovascular disease risk in women with diabetes?Am J Clin Nutr November 2004 vol. 80 no. 5 1194-1200.

[8] Vitamin E and Health. Harvard School of Public Health. Web. 2 Dec 2014.http://www.hsph.harvard.edu/nutritionsource/vitamin-e/

[9] Hancock, Robert D. Recent Patents on Vitamin C: Opportunities for Crop Improvement and Single-Step Biological Manufacture.Recent Patents on Food, Nutrition & Agriculture, 2009, 1, 39-49.

[10] Chen, Zhong et al. Increasing vitamin C content of plants through enhanced ascorbate recycling. Proc Natl Acad Sci U S A. 2003 Mar 18; 100(6): 3525–3530.Published online 2003 Mar 6. doi: 10.1073/pnas.0635176100

[11] Bagchi, Anamika. Extraction of Curcumin. Journal of Environmental Science, Toxicology and Food Technology.2319-2399. Volume 1, Issue 3 (Sep-Oct. 2012), PP 01-16.

[12] Turmeric Oleoreisin. Monograph, Additive: Food and Agricultural Organization of the United Nations. Web. 2 Dec 2014. http://www.fao.org/ag/agn/jecfa-additives/specs/Monograph1/Additive-484.pdf

[13] El-Adawi, Ayman E. Efficacy of Turmeric Powder Against 1,2 Dichlorethane-Induced Toxicity in Rats. Med. J . Cairo Univ., Vol. 76, No. 3, September: 495-502, 2008.

[14] Burgos-Moron, E et al. The dark side of curcumin. Letter to the Editor. Int. J. Cancer: 126, 1771–1775 (2010) VC 2009 UICC.

[15] Jäger, Ralf et al. Comparative absorption of curcumin formulations. Nutrition Journal 2014, 13:11 http://www.nutritionj.com/content/13/1/11. Web. 2 Dec, 2014.

[16] Antony B, Merina B, Iyer VS, Judy N, Lennertz K, Joyal S: A pilot cross-over study to evaluate human oral bioavailability of BCM-95CG (Biocurcumax), a novel bioenhanced preparation of curcumin. Indian J Pharm Sci 2008, 70(4):445–449.

[17] Shoba, G; Joy, D; Joseph, T; Majeed, M; Rajendran, R; Srinivas, P. S. Influence of piperine on the pharmacokinetics of curcumin in animals and human volunteers. Planta Med 1998, 64 (4), 353– 6.

[18] Barbecue Meat Chemicals: Grilling and Cancer. World health.net. May 31, 2005. Wb. Dec. 2, 2014.

http://www.worldhealth.net/news/barbecue_meat_chemicalsgrilling_and_ca
nc/
[19] Murkovic, M et al. Antioxidant spices reduce the formation of heterocyclic amines in fried meat.Zeitschrift für Lebensmitteluntersuchung und -Forschung A. November 1998, Volume 207, Issue 6, pp 477-480.DOI: 10.1007/s002170050364

CHAPTER 11

[1] Teng, Kim-Tiu. Modulation of obesity-induced inflammation by dietary fats: mechanisms and clinical evidence. Review: Nutrition Journal 2014, 13:12 http://www.nutritionj.com/content/13/1/12. Web. Dec 2, 2014.

[2] Duthey, Beatrice. Update on 2004 Tanna Saloni's Background Paper 6.11: Alzehimer Disease and other Dementias. 20 February 2013. World Health Organization. Web. 2 Dec. 2014.
http://www.who.int/medicines/areas/priority_medicines/BP6_11Alzheimer.
pdf.

[3] Libby, Peter. Inflammation and cardiovascular disease mechanisms. Am J Clin Nutr 2006;83(suppl):456S–60S.

CHAPTER 12

[1] Pahau, Helen et al. Cardiovascular disease is increased prior to onset of rheumatoid arthritis but not osteoarthritis: the population-based Nord-Trøndelag health study (HUNT). Arthritis Research & Therapy 2014, 16:R85 http://arthritis-research.com/content/16/2/R85.

[2] Fitzpatrick, FA. Cycooxygenase enzymes: regulation and function. Curr Pharm Des. 2004;10(6):577-88.

[3] Rouzer, Carol A. Cyclooxygenase: structural and functional insights. Journal of Lipid Research. April, 2009. 50; S29-S34.

[4] Tarleton State University. Anatomy. Inflammation. Benjamin Cummings. 2001. Web. Dec 2, 2014.
http://www.tarleton.edu/~anatomy/inflammation.html

[5] Robbins & Cotran's Pathological Basis of Disease. 8th Ed. Kumar V et al. (eds). Saunders Elselvier. Philadelphia (2010). With permission from the authors.

[6] Covas, Maria-Isabel. Review: Olive oil and the cardiovascular system. Pharmacological Research 55 (2007) 175–186.

[7] Suryakumar, Geetha and Gupta, Asheesh. Review: Medicinal and therapeutic potential of Sea Buckthorn (Hippophae rhamnoides L.). Journal of Ethnopharmacology 138 (2011) 268–278. `

[8] Gómez Candela, C et al. Importance of a balanced omega6/omega 3 ratio for the maintenance of health. Nutritional recommendations. Nutr Hosp. 2011;26(2):323-329

[9] Simopoulos, Artemis P. Mini-Review: The importance of the Omega-6/Omega-3 Fatty Acid Ratio in Cardiovascular Disease and Other Chronic Diseases. The Centre for Genetics, Nutrition and Health. Soc Exp Bio and Med. 2008. DOI: 10.3181/0711-MR-311

[10]Gómez Candela, C et al. Importance of a balanced omega6/omega 3 ratio for the maintenance of health. Nutritional recommendations. Nutr Hosp. 2011;26(2):326

[11] Tripoli, Elisa et al. The phenolic compounds of olive oil: structure, biological activity and beneficial effect on human health. Nutrition Research Reviews (2005), 18, 98-112. The Authors. 2005. DOI: 10.1079/NRR200495.

[12] Calder, Philip C. Omega-3 Fatty Acid and Inflammatory Processes. Nutrients 2010, 2, 355-374; doi: 10.3390/nu2030355.

CHAPTER 13

[1] Nitrates and Nitrites: TEACH Chemical Summary. United States Environmental Protection Agency. 22 May 2007. Web. 9 Dec 2014. http://www.epa.gov/teach/chem_summ/Nitrates_summary.pdf.

[2] Archer, Douglas L. Evidence that Ingested Nitrate and Nitrite Are Beneficial to Health. Journal of Food Protection, Vol. 65, No. 5, 2002, Pages 872–875.

[3] Sindelar, JJ and Milkowski, AL. Sodium Nitrite in Proceed Meat and Poultry Meats: A Review of Curing and Examining the Risk/Benefit of Its Use. American Meat Science Association, No. 3. Nov. 2011.

[4] Tong, Ming et al. Nitrosamine Exposure Causes Insulin Resistance Disease: Relavence to Type 2 Diabetes Mellitus, Non-Alcoholic Steatohepatitis, and Alzheimer's Disease. National Institute of Health Public Access. J Alzheimers Dis. 2009 ; 17(4): 827–844.

[5] Preservative use in processed meats: Licensee Guidance. NSW Food Authority. December 2009. Web. 9 Dec 2014. www.foodauthority.nsw.gov.au.

[6] Dietary fats, oils and cholesterol. Heart and Stroke Foundation. August 2012. Web. 9 Dec 2014. http://goo.gl/Xg81sx.

[7] Koller, Daniel et al. Effects of Oxidized Phospholipids on Gene Expression in RAW 264.7 Macrophages: A Microarray Study.

[8] He, L et al. Psoriasis decreases the anti-oxidation and anti-inflammation properties of high-density lipoprotein. Biochim Biophys Acta. 2014 Sep 18;1841(12):1709-1715. doi: 10.1016/j.bbalip.2014.09.008.

[9] Obradovic MM, et al. Interrelatedness between C-reactive protein and oxidized low-density lipoprotein.

[10] Davies, Kelvin JA. Oxidative Stress, Antioxidant Defences, and Damage Removal, Repair, and Replacement Systems. IUBMB Life, 50: 279-289, 2000. Clin Chem Lab Med. 2015 Jan 1;53(1):29-34. doi: 10.1515/cclm-2014-0590.

[11] Dr. Aubrey de Grey Transcript with Ann Wixon. The Future of Health Now 2012. Web. 9 Dec 2014. http://futureofhealth.s3.amazonaws.com/interviews/transcript/DeGrey.pdf

CHAPTER 14
[1] Pollan, Michael. Cooked: A Natural History of Transformation. Penguin Books, 2013. Print.
[2] Schardt, David. Slammin' Salmon - Farmed Salmon Under Fire. Nutrition Action Healthletter. June, 2004. Web. 8 Dec 2014. https://www.cspinet.org/nah/06_04/farmedsalmon.pdf.
[3] Consumer Factsheet on Perchlorinated Bisphenyls. National Primary Drinking Water Regulations. U.S. Environmental Protection Agency. May 14, 2009.
[4] Foran, JA et al. Risk-Based Consumption Advice for Farmed Atlantic and Wild Pacific Salmon Contaminated with Dioxins and Dioxin-like Compounds. Health Perspectives 113:552-556 (2005). DOI: 10.1289/ehp.7626.
[5] Hellerstein, Marc K. Carbohydrate-induced hypertriglyceridemia: modifying factors and implications for cardiovascular risk. Curr Opin Lipidol 13:33±40. 5 2002 Lippincott Williams & Wilkins.
[6] Soni, Himesh et al. A Recent Update of Botanicals for Wound Healing Activity. International Research Journal of Pharmacy. 2012, 3(3).
[7] Nevin, KG and Rajamohan, T. Effect of Topical Application of Virgin Coconut Oil on Skin Components and Antioxidant Status during Dermal Wound Healing in Young Rats. Skin Pharmacol Physiol 2010;23:290–297 DOI: 10.1159/000313516.
[8] Anitha, T. Medicinal Plants Used in Skin Protection. Asian Journal of Pharmaceutical and Clinical Research. Vol. 5, Suppl3, 2012.
[9] Mansor, T.S.T et al. Physicochemical properties of virgin coconut oil extracted from different processing methods. International Food Research Journal 19(3): 837-845 (2012).
[10] Dayrit, Conrado S. Coconut Oil: Atherogenic or Not? (What therefore causes Atherosclerosis?). Philippine Journal of Cardiology. July-September 2003, Vol 31, No. 3: 97-104.

CHAPTER 15
[1] Sauer, Abby C and Voss, Anne C. Improving Outcomes with Nutrition in Patients with Cancer. Abbott Nutrition. May 2012.
[2] Arends J, Bodoky G, Bozzetti F et al. ESPEN guidelines on enteral nutrition: non-surgical oncology. Clin, Nutr. 2006;25:245-259.
[3] REAL FOOD- Makaveli Motivation- Rich Piana- Phil Heath- Jay Cutler- Kali Muscle- Kai Greene. Rich Piana - Youtube Video. Oct. 29, 2014. https://www.youtube.com/watch?v=9KJFI1gfn_0.

[4] Coca-Cola's new ad: obesity 'concerns all of us' - video. The Guardian. January 15, 2013. Web. 9 Dec 2014. http://www.theguardian.com/business/video/2013/jan/15/coca-cola-ad-obesity-video.

CHAPTER 16

[1] Dietary fats, oils and cholesterol. Heart and Stroke Foundation. August, 2012. Web. 9 Dec 2014. http://goo.gl/3eTLCF.

[2] Gruère, GP and Rao, SR. A Review of International Labeling Policies of Genetically Modified Food to Evaluate India's Proposed Rule. AgBioForum, 10(1): 51-64. 2007.

[3] Mamur, S et al. Does potassium sorbate induce genotoxic or mutagenic effects in lymphocytes? Toxicol In Vitro. 2010 Apr;24(3):790-4. doi: 10.1016/j.tiv.2009.12.021.

[4] Proposal For Harmonised Classification and Labelling. CLH Report. November 2011. Germany. 9 Dec 2014. http://goo.gl/ysk7fT.

[5] Benbrook, Charles M. Impacts of genetically engineered crops on pesticide use in the U.S. — the first 16 years. Benbrook Environmental Sciences Europe 2012, 24:24.

[6] Choudhary, Nilesh et al. Isolation of Soy Lecithin From Soy Sludge, It's Standardization and Behavioural Study. Asian Journal of Pharmaceutical and Clinical Research. Vol 6, Issue 2, 2013.

[7] Kramer, Stanley. It's a Mad, Mad, Mad, Mad World. United Artists. November 7, 1963.

CHAPTER 17

[1] Smith, Jeffrey M. Genetic Roulette: The Gamble of Our Lives. The Institute for Responsible Technology. August, 2012.

[2] Wong, Jonathan et al. Grass-Fed versus Organic Dairy Production: Southeastern US Willingness to Pay. American Agricultural Economics Association Annual Meeting, Orlando, FL ,July 27-29, 2008. Web. 9 Dec 2014. http://ageconsearch.umn.edu/bitstream/6268/2/470124.pdf.

[3] Dhiman, T.R., G.R. Anand, et. al. "Conjugated linoleic acid content of milk from cows fed different diets." Journal of Dairy Science 82:10(1999): 2146-56.

CHAPTER 18

[1] Anjum, MI et al. Effect of Fresh Versus Oxidized Soybean Oil on Growth Peformance, Organs Weights And Meat Quality of Broiler Chicks. Pakistan Vet. J., 24(4): 2004.

[2] Chae, BJ. Effects of Feeding Rancid Rice Bran on Growth Performance and Chicken Meat Quality in Broiler Chicks. College of Animal Resources Si. Korea. 2001: 266-278.

[3] Garcia, M.D. et al. Hypocholesterolemic and Hepatoprotective Effects of "Triguero" Asparagus from Andalusia in Rats Fed a High Cholesterol Diet. Hindawi Publishing Corporation Evidence-Based Complementary and Alternative Medicine Volume 2012, Article ID 814752, 6 pages doi:10.1155/2012/814752.

[4] Okwari O.A et al. Anti-Hypercholesterolemic and Hepatoprotective effect of Aqueous Leaf Extract of Moringa oleifera in Rats fed with Thermoxidized Palm Oil Diet. OSR Journal of Pharmacy and Biological Sciences. Volume 8, Issue 2 (Nov.—Dec. 2013), PP 57-62.

[5] Singh, Harmeet. Hepatoprotective Activity of Turmeric and Garlic against 7-12, Dimethylbenzanthracene Induced Liver Damage in Wistar Albino Rats. European Journal of Medicinal Plants 1(4): 162-170, 2011.

[6] Pittler, WB et al. Artichoke leaf extract for treating hypercholesterolaemia (Review). John Wiley & Sons Publishing. 2009, Issue 4.

[7] Thompson Coon, JS et al. Herbs for serum cholesterol reduction: A systemic review. Peninsula Medical School, UK. June 2003. Vol. 52, No. 6.

[8] Your Guide to Lowering Your Cholesterol with TLC. U.S. Department of Health and Human Resources. NIH Pub No. 06-5235. Dec. 2005. Web. 10 Dec 2014.

[9] Low-Energy-Dense Foods and Weight Management: Cutting Calories While Controlling Hunger. Research to Practice Series, No. 5. Nat Center for Chron Dis Prev & Health Prom Div of Nut, Phys Act and Obesity. CDC. Web. 10 Dec 2014. http://www.cdc.gov/nccdphp/dnpa/nutrition/pdf/r2p_energy_density.pdf.

[10] Nina Cecile Øverby et al. Dietary fiber and the glycemic index: a background paper for the Nordic Nutrition Recommendations 2012. Food & Nutrition Research 2013. 57: 20709.

[11] Carroccio, Antonio et al. Chronic constipation and food intolerance: A model of proctitis causing constipation. Scandinavian Journal of Gastroenterology. 2005, Vol. 40, No. 1, Pages 33-42 (doi: 10.1080/00365520410009401).

[12] A. Carroccio and G. Iacono. Review article: chronic constipation and food hypersensitivity — an intriguing relationship. Alimentary Pharmacology & Therapeutics. Vol. 24, Issue 9. Pages 1295-1304. November 2006.

[13] Scalici, Calogero et al. Cow's Milk Intolerance and Chronic Constipation in Children. Aclinicaland Histology Study. Acta Pediatrica Mediterranea, 2005, 21: 85.

[14] Carroccio, Antonio et al. Case Report: Multiple food hypersensitivity as a cause of refractory chronic constipation in adults. Scandinavian Journal of Gastroenterology, 2006; 41: 498-504.

[15] Bhargava, Alok. Fiber Intakes and Anthropometric Measures are Predictors of Circulating Hormone, Triglyceride, and Cholesterol Concentrations in the Women's Health Trial. The Journal of Nutrition. 136: 2249–2254, 2006.

[16] Nilsson AC, et al. Including indigestible carbohydrates in the evening meal of healthy subjects improves glucose tolerance, lowers inflammatory markers, and increases satiety after a subsequent standardized breakfast. J Nutr. 2008;138:732-739.

[17] Pulses and Cardiovascular Disease. Pulse Canada. Web. 10 Dec 2014. http://goo.gl/YKKuIA.

[18] Carlson, Diana G. Glucosinolates in Crucifer Vegetables: Broccoli, Brussel's Sprouts, Cauliflower, Collards, Kale, Mustard Greens, and Kohlrabit. J. Amer. Soc. Hort. Sci 112(1):173-178. 1987.

[19] Schulick, Paul. Ginger: Common Spice and Wonder Drug. Third Edition. Herbal Free Press, Copyright 1996.

[20] Akhondzadeh, S et al. Salvia officinalis extract in the treatment of patients with mild to moderate Alzheimer's disease: a double blind, randomized and placebo-controlled trial. J Clin Pharm Ther. 2003 Feb;28(1):53-9.

[21] Perry, Nicolette S.L. et al. Salvia for dementia therapy: review of pharmacological activity and pilot tolerability clinical trial. Pharmacology, Biochemistry and Behavior 75 (2003) 651–659.

[22] Gounelle, H et al. Olive Oil and Blood Cholesterol Levels. American Journal of Clinical Nutrition. Vol. 10, February 1962.

[23] Cicerale, Sara et al. Biological Activities of Phenolic Compounds Present in Virgin Olive Oil. Int. J. Mol. Sci. 2010, 11, 458-479; doi:10.3390/ijms11020458.

[24] Zhang, Xianglan et al. Cruciferous vegetable consumption is associated with a reduced risk of total and cardiovascular disease mortality. Am J Clin Nutr 2011;94:240–6.

[25] Hyson, DA et al. Almonds and Almond Oil Have Similar Effects on Plasma Lipids and LDL Oxidation in Healthy Men and Women. J. Nutr. 132: 703–707, 2002.

[26] Abazarfard, Zohreh et al. The effect of almonds on anthropometric measurements and lipid profile in overweight and obese females in a weight reduction program: A randomized controlled clinical trial. J Res Med Sci. May 2014: 19(5) 457-464.

CHAPTER 19

[1] Brensing, Tess. Master of Science Thesis: Reduction of Heterocyclic Amine Formation in Beef By Surface Application of Spices. B.S., Kansas State University, 2009.

[2] Population Nutrient Intake Goals for Preventing Diet-Related Chronic Disease. Fish. World Health Organization. Web. Jan. 12, 2015.

http://www.who.int/nutrition/topics/5_population_nutrient/en/index13.html.
[3] Fish and Omega-3 Fatty Acids. The American Heart Association. May 14, 2014. Web. Jan 12, 2015.
http://www.heart.org/HEARTORG/GettingHealthy/NutritionCenter/Health yDietGoals/Fish-and-Omega-3-Fatty-Acids_UCM_303248_Article.jsp
[4] Kalueff, Allan V and Nutt, David J. Role of GABA in Anxiety and Depression. Depression & Anxiety 24:495–517 (2007).
[5] Final Assessment Report on Melissa officinalis., folium. European Medicines Agency; 14 May 2013. Web. 10 Dec 2014. http://goo.gl/v0B6Vh.

CHAPTER 20

[1] Plant Sterols and Blood Cholesterol Lowering. Food and Nutrition. Health Canada. Nov. 22, 2010. Web. Jan. 12, 2015. http://www.hc-sc.gc.ca/fn-an/label-etiquet/claims-reclam/assess-evalu/phytosterols-eng.php.
[2] Your Guide to Lowering Your Cholesterol with TLC. U.S. Department of Health and Human Resources. NIH Pub No. 06-5235. Dec. 2005. Web. 10 Dec 2014.
[3] Mayo Clinic Staff. Niacin can boost 'good' cholesterol. High Cholesterol. Mayo Clinic. April 12, 2014. Web. Jan. 20, 2015. http://www.mayoclinic.org/diseases-conditions/high-blood-cholesterol/in-depth/niacin/art-20046208
[4] Cheng, et al. Prolonged Fasting reduces IGF-1/PKA to promote hematopoietic stem cell-based regeneration and reverse immunosuppression. Cell Stem Cell. 2014 June 5; 14(6): 810–823. doi:10.1016/j.stem.2014.04.014.

About the Author

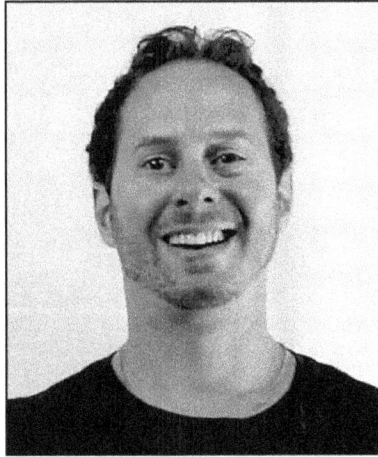

More important than his academic achievements, for over 30 years, Dr. Robert W. Horovitz, B.Sc., ND has been dreaming of helping people. Yes, literally since the age of 5. After earning his Bachelor of Science Degree at York University in 2003, with a focus in Molecular Biology and Organic Chemistry, he completed the Naturopathic Doctor program at The Canadian College of Naturopathic Medicine in Toronto, Ontario in 2008. In addition to several years of clinical practice, Robert has given thousands of combined presentations, trainings, consumer lectures, and keynotes; educating, inspiring, and learning from hundreds of combined health care professionals and leaders within the natural health industry, focusing on chronic disease and innovative natural health product distinctions.

www.ingramcontent.com/pod-product-compliance
Lightning Source LLC
Chambersburg PA
CBHW031504270326
41930CB00006B/244